Fitness M̶ for Weight L and S

How to Maximize Fitness Motivation, Weight Loss Motivation, Diet Motivation, Exercise Motivation, Workout Motivation, and Health Motivation

Version 1.0

By C. Townsend, M.A.

Legal Notice

Disclaimer

her physician for advice on whether to embark on the activities, physical, mental or otherwise, described herein.

Table of Contents

Introduction

Getting Started
With Fitness Motivation

Thank you for purchasing this book. I have written this guide with a single objective in mind—to help you become more healthy and fit by increasing your fitness motivation and consistency to the absolute maximum.

Motivation (short term and long term) is a major factor in determining your success in exercise, dieting, weight loss, weight maintenance, sports, and general health. Maximizing fitness motivation and consistency is an absolute necessity (and key solution) for highly successful weight loss achievers, fitness masters, and champion athletes.

If you are reading this, odds are this is not the first time you have entertained the thought of gaining control over your fitness motivation, weight, or physical fitness. You are intuitively aware that, with each passing day, month or year, the situation is not getting any better.

You may have tried to ignore it, become friends with it, be firm with it, go to war with it, and surrender to it. You may even have had minor victories. Yet, deep within, you know the pattern. You end up starting over, once again entertaining the thought of gaining control over your fitness and weight. What you want and need is an effective alternative to yo-yo dieting and occasional or sporadic exercising.

There are those without fitness motivation issues who have unconsciously and, by sheer accident, achieved long-term fitness and weight loss success. Ironically, they stumbled into the proven principles of lasting fitness motivation. They may appear to be the fortunate ones. But, if any life event or circumstance alters their unconscious achievement of fitness and weight loss, they too will suffer the consequences. In addition, they will have no idea or process by which they can consciously regain the needed fitness motivation and healthy habit consistency.

Fitness Motivation for Weight Loss, Exercise, and Sports is a simple yet effective solution for developing the habit of fitness motivation and consistency. If you will apply the information in this book, you can develop the knowledge and skills to identify and overcome your individual obstacles to developing the habits of regular exercise and healthy eating.

The multi-billion-dollar weight loss and fitness industry is brimming with tempting promises and easy solutions that tout miracles of rapid weight loss and instant fitness. This book has evolved from many years of observation with clients, research, and participation. During this time, it became clear to me that deprivation diets, unproven supplements, and over-hyped exercise gadgets are not helpful for those of us who want sustainable fitness and weight loss. If they were, 65% of the population would not be overweight or dealing with the consequences of obesity.

I came to understand that if your goal is fitness, weight loss, or weight management—you really need a *simple yet innovative solution that will actually help you* _maintain_ *a healthy diet and regular exercise as part of your lifestyle.*

Diet and exercise are essential ingredients in fitness and weight loss. Make no mistake about it, successful weight loss and fitness improvement require some level of adjustment in your diet and physical activity. But, there is more to it. This guide will provide you with the critical missing elements to fitness motivation success.

What You Will Find in This Guide

This book contains a simple, proven method for fitness motivation and long-term fitness success. The objectives of this how-to guide are as follows:

1. Provide a fitness motivation method and process that will help you develop the fitness habit for life-long success in weight management and exercise consistency.

2. Provide a fitness motivation method and process that is easy for you to implement and maintain.

To achieve the goals of this guide--I have included practical solutions, proven scientific principles, concise instructions, effective tools, and innovative concepts.

This book contains the following eleven chapters:

Chapter 1: Reject Fitness and Weight Loss Fantasies

How to Get Your Money's Worth From This Book

You should not read this guide and put it aside once you are done. I am your advisor, and this guide is the beginning of a two-way conversation between you, who wants to become a more consistent exerciser and healthy eater by maximizing your fitness motivation, and me, who is providing the essential information that will help you achieve your goal.

I believe that this guide is unlike any other ever published on the subject of motivation for fitness, weight loss, dieting, and exercise. By breaking down all of the key components of motivation and relying on science and the experience of current and past clients—this guide can help you maximize your fitness motivation within a short period of time.

For starters, I suggest you browse through the book to get a conceptual view of its contents and direction. From there, you should study each chapter. The chapters are in a specific order to build your fitness motivation one step at a time. After reading each chapter--you should reflect, make highlights, and take notes.

A Few Words About Me and My Role in Your Life

As your fitness motivation advisor, please allow me to summarize my background and experience.

My specialty is the Psychology of exercise and nutrition. I have a Master's degree in exercise and sports psychology. Over the last few years, I have focused on creating a simple and practical blueprint for developing a *sustainable fitness motivation habit* to help people achieve and maintain fitness and weight loss success.

I continue to devour any information I can find on fitness motivation and the psychology of fitness. In this guide, you will find effective solutions for developing your fitness motivation, diet habits, and exercise habits. I will not mislead you regarding what it really takes to overcome internal obstacles to lasting fitness. Many people out there will. Do not let them!

Okay, enough about that—now let's get started on your fitness motivation training.

Chapter 1

Reject Fitness and Weight Loss Fantasies

After developing sufficient motivation, most people assume that taking immediate action will automatically lead to fitness and weight loss success. Unfortunately, many highly motivated, eager people fail to take the _correct_ actions. They rush headlong down the wrong path, choosing to take misguided and temporary actions that lead to short-term results. Typically, they fail to achieve lasting results because they have become victims of _fitness and weight loss fantasies._

Weight loss fantasies are powerful. All that is required is a high susceptibility to the idea of a quick, easy, simple, magical cure for being unfit or overweight. These fantasies are accompanied by exaggerated promises of amazing results and are only temporary fixes.

Traveling the weight loss fantasy road will not lead to success. Weight loss and fitness comes from letting go of the fantasy thoughts and actions. If you buy into the fantasies, you will simply be taking a tour of an imaginary *fitness fantasyland.*

Don't undermine your fitness motivation by taking the wrong actions or being influenced by fantasy fitness ideas. Let's review some very common fitness and weight loss misconceptions. By understanding these failed strategies, you will be able to ignore them—and focus on using your growing motivation to make real progress toward fitness and weight loss success.

Harboring Delusions

Harboring delusions about weight loss or fitness is very common. In fact, this flawed fitness and weight loss strategy is one of the oldest and most beloved attractions in the imaginary fitness fantasyland. We've all experienced those familiar delusions of grandeur. It's where the fun, adventure, and fantasy begin. It's a mirror-lined maze that reflects whatever you desire.

The flawed strategy of harboring delusions (or believing illusions) appeals to unrealistic self-images and expectations of quick fixes. It captivates the mind and emotions. It opens up the consciousness to the possibility of amazing results and unbelievable claims.

It is the perfect setup for a fitness fantasyland experience.

The most effective counter to fitness and weight loss delusions is knowledge. My job (and the job of this guide) is to provide you with the right knowledge to effectively avoid and counter fallacies that can undermine your fitness and weight loss success.

The Great Promise: Quick & Easy

The great promise is all about *quick and easy* benefits. Desperate individuals sometimes find themselves looking for the "big secret" and its promise of a magical cure for being overweight and unfit.

Some might think that the expectation of a drastic, quick, and easy weight loss is questionable, but they want to believe. The promise of losing fifty pounds---quicker and easier than ever before—and without doing ab crunches or giving up french fries will appeal to most people.

But, here's the reality: *Exaggerated declarations and promises that seem phenomenal, purporting to be quick and easy, are usually tip offs that you are being lured out of reality and into fitness fantasyland.* If the outlandish claims were true, 65% of Americans would not be overweight or obese.

1-800-SuckerMeNow

This silly little fitness and weight loss fallacy comes complete with celebrities. They smile and twirl, turning left, then right and back again, filling you with envy for their seemingly wonderful happy lives and drop-dead gorgeous bodies. The fact that they are also sexy is a bonus.

This celebrity-endorsed fitness fantasy operates even in the wee hours of the night, with operators standing by. Sometimes you will see distinguished people sporting white lab coats and pens in their breast pocket, portraying the role of a health care professional. Of course, all of these amazing products are only available exclusively and for a limited time only.

Unfortunately, for some of us--we watch far too much television. Infomercials are not the most reliable medium for receiving the proper knowledge or advice on fitness or weight loss. First and foremost, their primary goal is to relieve you of your money. Any actual physical benefit given to you is a bonus. *Remember: The endorsing celebrities and actor/doctors are paid.* And yes, the enthusiastic audience members are paid too.

At the very least, do your homework before calling 1-800-SUCKERMENOW, even if callers within the next ten minutes get a free bonus!

Miracle Diet

The Miracle Diet is like a water ride at an amusement park. It has individual boats that glide in a leisurely manner around and around in a circle. Each one has a catchy little name painted on its side, like Vinegar, Cabbage, and Grapefruit Juice! Miracle and fad diets pre-date your grandmother's youth. Prior to the current weight loss industry boom, these diets were all the rage.

If miracle or fad diets were so effective, why are so many of our grandmothers, mothers, and aunts overweight? It's because these so-called miracle diets are unhealthy and produce minimal results that are temporary at best. The minute you return to "normal" eating, you will regain the weight. You would have to remain on these diets for the rest of your life. Just how much do you like cabbage?

Super Supplement

So-called super supplements are one of the fastest growing segments of the nutrition industry. They are super-stimulating and energizing. Typically they contain vitamins, minerals, herbs, and some form of caffeine all rolled into one. These high-energy supplements will cause your metabolism to speed up and promise outrageous benefits like causing fat cells to shrink.

Taking supplements is serious and you should be just as careful with supplements as you are with prescription drugs. Millions of Americans are purchasing an over-the-counter supplement without truly understanding its effect on their physiology. And if one doesn't work, they stop it and start taking a different one they heard about on television, read about in a magazine, or were urged to take by a friend, family member, or co-worker.

Using a diet supplement to alter metabolism or "shrink fat cells" is not recommended by any "credible" medical professional. It can be medically dangerous. Unlike prescription medications, supplements are not regulated by the Food and Drug Administration.

Interactions among various supplements may lead you to the doctor's office or emergency room. Not all supplements are to be avoided, but it is always prudent to be an informed user and discuss any supplements with your doctor.

Good Foods, Bad Foods

Any food (in moderation) is not inherently good or bad. Carbohydrates, fat, protein, and even the occasional treat can occupy a place in your healthy and fit lifestyle. Too much of anything generally produces an imbalance that may be unhealthy.

Make food selections with overall health and balance as a primary focus, rather than placing an extreme "all or nothing" judgment value on any particular food or food group. Moderation and balance are real-world lifestyle choices that lead to improved motivation, fitness, and lasting weight loss.

New Fads

I've counseled many clients who can be described as weight loss or fitness "fad fanatics." They simply can't resist the latest, hottest new thing. There are quick-and-easy diet plans, amazing new non-exercise exercise programs, and simple fat-busting power shakes, bars, and topical creams.

Fads are seen as new, trendy, fashionable, and in vogue. What that really means is that the product is hyped, aggressively marketed, and typically unproven. Being a fad does not validate the science or the effectiveness of a fitness or weight loss product. Fads, by their very nature, come and go. Do not follow the fitness fad crowd and you will be on your way to personal weight loss and fitness success.

Pseudoscience

Every tabloid-style media outlet or infomercial touts the newest or latest scientific weight loss breakthrough. It's often difficult to distinguish credible science from pseudoscience.

Hint: If there ever is an honest scientific weight loss breakthrough, you won't have to wait to see it on the cover of a supermarket tabloid magazine. It will be the lead story on the evening news and every television and radio talk show. Do not act upon these pseudoscience breakthroughs. They are for entertainment purposes only.

Magic Gadgets

Have you or someone you know ever purchased a fitness gadget—such as a miraculous tummy flattening machine?

When you fall prey to unproven fitness gadgets—you are often buying into the false notion of "spot reduction." There is no such thing as losing fat in one specific spot on your body, such as your tummy or thighs.

Gadgets that promise to "blast fat" from one area of your body are bogus! Honestly, does it even sound reasonable? Spot reduction is a myth. You may be able to tone your muscles, but the fat cells in your stomach are there for life. With proper weight loss, you can reduce the size of the fat cells but they do not disappear and you can't "zap or shake" them away.

Fitness and Weight Loss Reality

The primary rule of fitness and weight loss reality is that you must not allow your mind to be influenced by fitness fantasyland. The fitness misconceptions highlighted in this chapter can be enticing and alluring when packaged and marketed in the right way. However, these money-sucking fantasy feeders will only provide false hope and temporary motivation, which will ultimately lead to short-term results and eventual failure.

You don't have to fall into this trap. If you have already done so, do not despair. Many who achieve long term fitness and weight loss success have been where you are. It is an easy cycle to fall into. Billions of dollars are specifically targeted to lure you into the promises of quick and easy fixes.

You are motivated to get fit and lose weight. This is truly powerful! You will stop the fitness and weight loss "merry-go-round" if you are willing to direct your motivation and enthusiasm toward real solutions and proven strategies.

Please don't undermine your fitness motivation energy by rushing into "random and incorrect" actions. Instead, focus on gaining the proper knowledge that will allow you to take *"specific and correct"* actions for continuous improvement, consistent motivation, and lasting results.

Chapter 2

Embrace Natural Laws of Weight Loss and Fitness

There is a core knowledge that must accompany your motivation and precede your action. This is not just *any* knowledge. This is the *proper* knowledge that will lead to fitness, weight loss, and a healthy lifestyle.

In order to make the proper decisions, you must understand and accept the *natural laws* of weight loss and fitness. These proven natural laws are science-based and have been validated through consistent results. Understanding these key principles will keep you rooted in reality and away from fitness fantasyland.

Any fitness or weight loss program must be grounded in fundamental natural laws in order to achieve long-term success and sustainable results. These basics embrace the natural physiology and psychology of fitness and weight loss.

The most significant law for weight loss is **Energy Balance**: The balance between energy taken in, generally by food and drink, and energy expended.

Metabolism, the process by which your body converts food into energy that is needed to sustain itself, is affected by three distinct but critical elements: **RMR**—resting metabolic rate, **TEF**—thermic effect of food, and **TEA**—thermic effect of activity. *The greatest opportunity to positively affect metabolism is through TEA.*

Proper **Nutrition** is essential to supply the appropriate daily intake of nutrients, minerals, and vitamins that the body requires to support its vital functions and perform at its peak.

Physical Activity and exercise is critical to effective weight loss, physical fitness, and overall health.

Lifestyle behaviors and environment can have a significant impact on health and weight management.

Energy Balance

Calories are the measurement units of energy balance. They measure the potential heat energy in the food and drink we consume. Calories represent fuel that the body needs to function.

Daily food intake is the consumption of calories. Daily activities and the body's basic physiological tasks expend or use calories.

The human body functions on a supply and demand system. If the daily consumption of calories meets the body's demand--the excess calories are stored for future use, in the form of fat. The reserves of stored fat are available for energy usage when the body's demand for calories exceeds the daily calorie consumption.

Weight gain is the result of excess consumption and storage of calories within the body. When calorie intake exceeds calorie expenditure, the result is weight gain. When calorie expenditure exceeds calorie intake, the result is weight loss. When calories taken in equal the calories expended, weight is maintained.

3,500 calories is equal to one pound. If you consume 3,500 *more* calories than you burn over a period of time—you will gain one pound. If you consumer 3,500 *less* calories than you burn over a period of time—you will lose one pound.

Your weight and management of your weight is dependent upon this one simple principle. It's simply the balancing of *"calories in and calories out."*

Metabolism

The breakdown of food and its transformation into energy is a function of the body's metabolism process—and there are three key elements of your metabolism.

1. **Resting Metabolic Rate (RMR):** The amount of energy (calories) that supports essential body functions, such as the cardio-respiratory system, and the body at rest. RMR represents 65% of daily metabolism or calories burned for the average adult.

2. **Thermic Effect of Food (TEF):** The amount of energy (calories) that supports digestion, absorption, and the metabolism of food. This is not the calories of the food, but only the energy the body actually uses to digest and process food in your body. TEF represents 10% of daily calories burned for the average adult.

3. **Thermic Effect of Activity (TEA):** The amount of additional energy (calories) due to physical activity. TEA represents 25% of daily calories burned for the average adult.

Your RMR (Resting Metabolic Rate) is determined by genetics, age, weight, gender, and muscle mass. The only elements that you can affect are weight and muscle mass.

Your body weight has a significant impact on your metabolism. The more you weigh, the higher your metabolism will be (all other things being equal). Consequently--as you lose weight, your metabolism will slow down because your body has to burn less calories to maintain a lower weight.

The greatest opportunity to improve your metabolism in a healthy way is by manipulating the TEA (Thermic Effect of Activity) element of your metabolism (through increased activity and exercise). Athletes and highly active individuals have a higher functioning metabolism because they consistently burn more calories and have higher muscle mass ratio due to higher physical activity levels.

The ability to significantly increase your metabolism by manipulating TEF (Thermic Effect of Food) is negligible. If you are already overweight— the bottom line is that you must increase your physical activity, and/or muscle ratio if you want to boost your metabolism.

Nutrition

Nutrition is the study of nutrients in food and their function as nourishment for the body. Forty-plus specific nutrients satisfy three basic functions—the need for energy, the need for tissue growth and repair, and the need to regulate metabolic function.

Nutrients are critical to the processes of digestion, absorption, metabolism, storage, and excretion. The six categories of nutrients are as follows:

1. Water

2. Vitamins

3. Minerals

4. Protein

5. Carbohydrates

6. Fat

Water

Water is as essential as oxygen in sustaining life. It is often easy to forget the importance of water, but it is critical for all body functions. Water supports proper cell function. It transports nutrients to the cells and removes cell waste. Water is also important for body temperature regulation.

Vitamins

Vitamins are essential organic substances that support body functions. They promote energy production, growth, maintenance, and repair. Small quantities of vitamins aid in human nutrition and metabolism. It is important that the nutrition consumed contain these essential substances, because the body can't manufacture them. Vitamins can't be used for fuel, because they have no caloric content.

Minerals

Minerals are inorganic substances important for healthy nutrition. They support the proper maintenance of vital body functions and processes such as the regulation of the heartbeat, transportation of oxygen to each cell, and the formation of hemoglobin—an essential protein in red blood cells, the healthy development of teeth and bones, and muscle contraction.

Protein

Protein is one of the three main macronutrients. Proteins contain carbon, oxygen, hydrogen, and nitrogen. These are important for the development and maintenance of the brain, muscles, skin, hair--and for the tissue that connects and supports body structure.

Proteins regulate body processes, such as water balance, with the production of enzymes and hormones. They play a vital role in the body's immune system--as critical components of antibodies, which fight foreign organisms and promote resistance to disease.

Proteins are one of the calorie nutrients. They supply fuel (energy) for the body.

1 gram of protein = 4 calories.

Carbohydrates

Carbohydrates are one of the three macronutrients. They are organic substances containing compounds of carbon, hydrogen, and oxygen.

Carbohydrates are the most important source of energy for your body. Your digestive system changes carbohydrates into glucose (blood sugar). Your body uses this sugar for energy for your cells, tissues and organs.

There are simple carbohydrates (which supply and burn energy quickly) and complex carbohydrates (which supply and burn energy more slowly).

1 gram of carbohydrates = 4 calories.

Fat

Fat is one of the three main macronutrients. There are many different kinds of fats, but each is a variation on the same chemical structure.

Fats are essential for good health. Fats play a vital role in maintaining healthy skin and hair, insulating body organs against shock, maintaining body temperature, and promoting healthy cell function. Fat also serves as a useful buffer against a host of diseases.

Fat serve both as an energy source for the body--and as a storage for energy in excess of what the body needs immediately. Because fat is a concentrated energy source, it contains more than twice the calories of protein and carbohydrates.

1 gram of fat = 9 calories.

Physical Activity

Physical activity centers on movement. It is important to engage in adequate physical activity in order to achieve fitness and lasting weight loss.

The two types of physical activity are *primary* and *supplemental.* Primary exercise is naturally occurring physical activity that is generally unplanned, unstructured, and spontaneous (such as playing with kids or having to jog to make it to an important meeting or class on time). Supplemental exercise is planned and more structured (such as planned jogging, swimming, strength training, yoga, etc).

Lifestyle

It is important to align your thoughts, behaviors, environment, and goals to effectively support successful achievement and maintenance of your desired fitness level and weight target.

With each successive step of your fitness or weight loss program, you move toward the development of healthier *habits* that will lead to a *fitness lifestyle.*

Your motivation *and* readiness for change are both important factors in determining whether or not you will reach your fitness goals.

Customization of any knowledge or program is also very important for fitness and weight loss success. Your fitness or weight loss program must meet your specific and unique needs and lifestyle requirements. One size does not fit all.

I encourage you to embrace all of the natural laws of fitness and weight loss! Commit to staying connected to reality and avoiding fitness fantasyland.

By respecting the scientific truth of the energy balance process—and the role that metabolism, nutrition, physical activity, and lifestyle play in achieving your fitness goals—you will have the knowledge and confidence to maintain motivation for consistent action and long term fitness and weight loss success.

Chapter 3

Take Charge of Your Fitness

If you live in Buffalo, New York, and intend to drive eighteen hours to Orlando, Florida, you may know that you will have to drive south. You may even be aware that your journey will take you through Pennsylvania, West Virginia, Virginia, North and South Carolina, and Georgia before you even reach the state of Florida.

Without GPS, a map, or directions of any kind, you could simply start driving south and maybe, eventually, reach your destination. It would be adventurous, but is that really what you want or need to do?

Having motivation and the general knowledge of north, east, south, and west is not enough. You must take charge of this journey.

It is the same with your fitness and weight management. You must take charge! Success requires your willingness to take charge of your behavior and actions so that you can actively manage the process that will lead to your destination of fitness and lasting weight loss.

Honest Assessment

Taking charge starts with taking stock of yourself and your unique and current situation. This must be an honest and thorough personal assessment, but without any judgment. You simply want to be objective and accurate about where you are from a fitness perspective--so that you can develop the right knowledge, goals, mental programming, and action plan for long-term success.

What is going on in your life that affects your fitness and weight? How does your body really look? Be honest about your body. At this point, what goals can realistically be set to move you toward fitness and your target weight?

Gaining a deeper understanding of your motivation, fears, strengths, weaknesses, and unique fitness personality is a proven and effective strategy for developing a plan that will inspire you to stick with it—develop the fitness habit—and maintain a fitness lifestyle.

Seize the Opportunity

We've all had moments in our lives when we are excited about something new—a change or an up-coming event. Yet, at the same time--we are filled with anxiety, doubt, and maybe even fear--because we are not certain of how or where to begin.

Sometimes, we are not sure how to get started with our fitness program. In that precise moment of uncertainty or indecision--you can either allow the excitement to propel you forward, or you can concede and allow the "status quo" of not taking action to continue.

The daily moments of key decision-making are crucial to your fitness motivation and success. You must acknowledge the power of these *"daily decision points"* as they are truly defining moments. The daily decision points are a gift and opportunity to move forward toward your improved fitness--or they can be an excuse to slide backward toward being more overweight and unhealthy.

It's your choice. You have the power! Seize the opportunity to *take charge of your fitness and health by simply making your daily decision points work for you* and not against you.

Assume Full Responsibility

Taking charge is great for jumpstarting your fitness motivation. When you take charge *and accept full responsibility* for your fitness without excuses—you will be more self-directed, self-reliant, and consistent in your actions and achievements. Assuming full responsibility for your fitness motivation will help you *maintain your fitness motivation.*

I encourage you to enlist others to help you. Positive and knowledgeable supporters can contribute tremendously to your motivation, fitness success, and weight loss accomplishments. However, you must ultimately play the central role in your own fitness and weight loss success.

Be bold and proud in assuming full responsibility for all of your results as you start your fitness program. Don't be afraid to share your successes and failures with your core supporters. You will often gain insights and inspiration from others.

Use your growing *knowledge and confidence* to assess results constantly, so that you can quickly correct mistakes. The motivating power of consistent improvement and results will eventually override and eliminate fear if you are willing to *take full responsibility for your success!*

Chapter 4

Commit To Your Fitness Lifestyle

Once you have made the decision to take responsibility for your fitness and weight loss—does this mean that you are committed?

The assumption of commitment by way of responsibility is a mistaken notion that many people accept. My goal is to help you become a *fitness motivation master*, so you must learn and internalize the fact that taking charge and accepting responsibility are crucial steps along your path to fitness success. You must also learn that taking charge and accepting responsibility are *not* the same as commitment.

Think of those instances in your life when you have seen someone volunteer to take charge or accept responsibility for something that, in the end, did not achieve the desired results. Maybe they began extremely gung-ho, yet somewhere along the line their motivation, enthusiasm, and energy faded and their effectiveness suffered. There are even those who have volunteered to take charge and who never show up! Something occurred between the time they made the decision to accept responsibility and the time it came to execute.

After you have accepted responsibility for your fitness, weight loss, and health--*it is time to make a conscious <u>commitment</u> to the fitness lifestyle*!

Commitment

Commitment is a state or quality of dedication. To be committed is to be obligated to something and willing to give 100%---not 80 or 90%--but, 100% focus and effort.

You must *commit fully* to the fitness lifestyle if you want to maximize your fitness motivation and physical results.

For fitness motivation masters, commitment is expressed as a conviction. For those lacking sufficient belief, commitment is typically expressed as a "wish" or "hope."

Most people don't make strong decisions or declarations. They state weak preferences. Preferences can be altered, ignored, or changed. Preferences are exceptionally vulnerable to excuses, adverse challenges, or circumstances.

You must "go all out" to truly separate yourself from the crowd. A decisive commitment is one where you leave no doubt about your conviction and future actions.

In the last chapter, we discussed taking charge and accepting responsibility. Now that you know that you are in charge of your fitness success---it is imperative that you fully commit to achieving it. Commitment is vitally important for anyone who wants to achieve a significant goal. A firm commitment makes fitness motivation easier and more sustainable.

Practice demonstrating commitment regularly. The best way to do this is to invest time, resources, and energy into the behaviors and activities that will deliver the desired results in fitness and weight loss. Stop investing in activities, things, or people that do not result in consistent progress toward your fitness and weight loss goals.

Keep in mind that commitment does not guarantee constant success. Fitness motivation masters may fail along the way to success, but they do not make excuses (remember, you must accept responsibility). You may occasionally falter in your journey to success, but you will learn to identify the true reasons for progress impairment—and you will learn to take immediate steps to correct bad decisions and behavioral mistakes.

For most people--real commitment is simple in principle, but hard to put into practice. For starters, I suggest you just commit that *you will not give up*—and that *you will persist* in gaining the knowledge, motivation, support, and tools to reach your fitness and weight loss goals. I've witnessed many clients experience a breakthrough in their fitness and weight loss, once they made a *no-excuse commitment to success!*

Success in fitness or weight loss does not often come immediately or even on the first try, but a commitment to the process will prevent you from "dropping out" of the process—which will ultimately lead to you achieving your goals faster.

The Fitness Lifestyle

The fitness lifestyle is *the enjoyable pursuit of optimum health and physical performance.* A fitness lifestyle fuels and maximizes your fitness motivation.

To live a fitness lifestyle you must commit to move beyond temporary fitness or weight loss solutions. You must commit to developing personal habits that support a fitness lifestyle and physical transformation. If you are unwilling to commit to a fitness lifestyle, you will be unwilling to make the choices and decisions needed to sustain fitness motivation and lasting physical results.

Any weight loss strategy that focuses *only* on weight loss will eventually fail. By committing to a fitness lifestyle, you will automatically lose weight. More importantly, you will finally keep it off. Fitness motivation masters happily embrace this fact. Conversely, yo-yo dieters and sporadic fitness enthusiasts consistently fail to accept the fact that *commitment to the fitness lifestyle is the most successful path to fitness and permanent weight loss.*

For the purpose of achieving fitness and weight loss success, there are two major components of the fitness lifestyle.

1. Effective management of your diet.

2. Effective management of your physical activity.

Below are the seven consistent behaviors of fitness motivation masters based on my observation and study of clients who have successfully achieved their target fitness and weight loss goals—and maintained their goals for more than one year.

1. Resolve and purpose (commitment).

2. Positive "can-do" attitude.

3. Healthy eating habits.

4. Active lifestyle.

5. Regular results tracking.

6. Willingness to accept full responsibility for success and failure.

7. Consistently seeking more knowledge on fitness and weight management.

Four Stages of Change

According to most psychological studies and journals, there are four stages of change: pre-contemplation, contemplation, preparation, and maintenance. Understanding these four stages of change, will help you monitor and manage your fitness motivation for the successful attainment of your physical goals.

Stage 1: Pre-contemplation

In this stage, there is no awareness or intention to change. There can be denial or pessimism about the ability to change. Sometimes it reveals itself in a "What's the point?" attitude.

Stage 2: Contemplation

This is the stage of change where many well-intentioned dieters and fitness enthusiasts remain stuck. They understand the value of making changes to their diet or activity routines. And, to some degree, they desire to make the change. Yet they waver between getting ready to make a change and actually making a consistent commitment and effort to change.

They may continually weigh the costs of change—effort, finances, time, effectiveness, benefits, and the effect on others. Sometimes this continuous "analysis paralysis" is used as psychological distraction from the need to accept full responsibility--or from the fear of short-term failure.

Stage 3: Preparation

Committing to a fitness lifestyle is the start of the preparation stage. In the preparation stage, the process of changing behavior begins. There is the beginning of effective actions (reducing calories, increasing physical activity, making healthier food choices, and an awareness of the importance of energy balancing).

This stage represents a significant step. It indicates that you are willing to commit the necessary time and energy toward achieving lasting change.

Stage 4: Maintenance

Fitness lifestyle maintenance and the development of sustainable habits is the goal of the fourth stage. In addition to physical results and success—this stage represents psychological transformation and freedom. Once you reach this stage, you will be a fitness motivation master!

Chapter 5

The MotivateFit™ Method

The MotivateFit™ Method is a simple, but powerful process for effectively customizing, strengthening, and managing your fitness motivation for short-term and long-term fitness and weight loss success.

The MotivateFit Method increases your fitness motivation by teaching you how to develop, integrate, and sustain the critical skills required to maximize your motivation and habits for fitness and weight loss.

Any knowledge, plan, resource, action, or skill utilized for the benefit of your personal fitness and weight loss is a *MotivateFit element*. It is the combination and consistent application of these crucial MotiveFit elements that will create your *personal MotivateFit Method*.

The five elements of the The MotivateFit Method include:

1. **Fitness Knowledge** (you must first acquire the correct information for success).

2. **Fitness Planning** (you must take the time to plan for success).

3. **Fitness Resources** (you must have the right tools and support for success).

4. **Fitness Actions** (you must take small consistent actions and adjust based on results).

5. **Fitness Skills** (you must continue to hone your motivation, exercise program, and diet skills).

The following flow chart summarizes The MotivateFit Method.

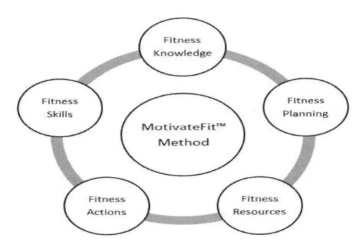

If you are lacking fitness motivation, it is because your MotivateFit elements are not individually strong—or your MotivateFit elements are not collectively in balance.

The MotivateFit Method in practical daily application is demonstrated by the *continuous and balanced progression of all MotivateFit elements*, which results in consistent improvement of your mental fitness (motivation) and physical fitness.

The key to developing sustainable fitness motivation is to stop looking for one singular or "secret" solution. The reality is that sustainable motivation and effective habits for fitness, exercise, and diet are developed by leveraging the five distinct, but interconnected solutions of the MotivatFit Method.

Focus on consistent improvement from day-to-day—avoid fitness fantasyland and trying to do too much too soon—and you will be on your way to properly using the MotivateFit Method for lasting success!

What Is Motivation?

The starting point for all achievement is motivation. Without sufficient motivation, you will not take that crucial first step toward success.

Motivation is literally the desire to do something. It's the difference between wanting to jump out of bed at the crack of dawn because you can't wait to start your workout—versus wanting to hit the snooze button.

Motivation requires emotion. Knowing something isn't enough to cause change. You must *feel* something emotionally, mentally, and physically that causes you to want and need the result you are seeking.

The term motivation describes *why* a person does something. Motivation is what causes us to act, whether it is eating something to satisfy our hunger or reading a book to gain knowledge.

Motives are those things that motivate us. Motives are the "whys" of behavior--the needs or wants that drive our actions and explain what we do. We can't actually observe the motives of others, but we can infer motives based on the behavior we observe in others.

Motivation is an essential element in setting and attaining goals—and research shows that you can influence and increase your own levels of motivation. The more you exercise your motivation--the more powerful it will become.

MotivateFit students view motivation as a skill that (like any other skill) can be improved with the proper knowledge and practice.

The Science of Motivation

Motivation is a process that initiates, guides, and maintains goal-oriented behaviors. Motivation can be divided into two types: intrinsic (internal) motivation and extrinsic (external) motivation.

Intrinsic motivation refers to motivation that is driven by an interest or enjoyment in the task itself, and exists within the individual rather than relying on external pressures or desires. People who are intrinsically motivated to succeed are naturally more enthusiastic about their fitness activities.

You are intrinsically motivated if you display the following three traits:

1. Belief that you have (or can develop) the skills to reach your goals.

2. Commitment to learning and mastering the required skills to reach your goals.

3. Acceptance of your power to influence your results and success.

Extrinsic motivation comes from outside of the individual. Extrinsic motivators include rewards, for exhibiting the desired behavior—and punishment, for not exhibiting the desired behavior.

I recommend using both intrinsic and extrinsic motivation methods to improve your fitness motivation and fitness habits.

In my own personal experience, I have found that I am most motivated when anchored by intrinsic motivational factors. From there, I identify compelling external motivational factors that will increase my total motivation. This dual approach to "motivation flexing" is particularly helpful in getting me past any initial procrastination related to a new goal or challenge.

If you are not motivated to take action on your most important goals—you should start with asking yourself, "why am I not motivated?"

Is it that you are not sure what you really want? Is it that you don't really want the reward? Is it that you believe the work required to achieve your fitness goal is too difficult? Is your fitness goal or objective in conflict with another goal or personal value? Do you doubt that you have "what it takes" to achieve your fitness goal?

Take the time to identify and understand the intrinsic and extrinsic motivators that will drive you to achieve your significant fitness and weight loss goals. Intimate knowledge of your key motivators will provide constant energy.

One of my favorite motivation sayings to MotivateFit students is this: *"you must be mindful before you can be motivated."* This means that it's always worth taking a timeout to assess your *motivation gaps* if you find that you are procrastinating or not feeling eager to take consistent action toward your fitness and health goals.

If you are not motivated—trust me, there is a logical reason for it. True, you may not know what that reason is—but, your mind is fighting against you for some reason that (if identified) can be addressed and overcome.

A conflict between your mind and your goals will weaken your fitness motivation and ability to reach your goals. To optimize your fitness habits, you must actively engage and hone your motivation. You can start by making sure you always have consistent alignment between your mind, fitness goals, and personal values.

Motivation Methods

The following solutions can help stimulate, increase, and maintain your motivation for fitness, exercise, dieting, and health. Use the motivation methods that work best for you and don't hesitate to try new solutions, or discard a solution if it's not working for you.

Goals

You can't achieve something if you don't know what you are trying to achieve! You must learn how to set and achieve goals if you want to develop your fitness and weight loss skills.

It is much easier to maintain motivation if the process of managing your goals is a regular and enjoyable activity in your life. By regular, I mean you should be reviewing and thinking about your big, inspiring fitness goals on a daily basis!

Goal setting provides instant benefits because it immediately focuses your brainpower on a specific outcome. Conversely, having no goals or unclear goals hinders motivation and power because your brain is more scattered and less focused.

The daily management of your fitness goals and activities will be easier and more effective if you use the MotivateFit process.

Music

Music is a great tool for stimulating and maintaining your motivation to give 100% to an exercise session. I find that music helps me enter the "zone" or peak performance state of mind—which increases my overall mental focus, motivation, and results.

Music can make any activity seem more enjoyable, creative, and fulfilling.

Nearly all champion athletes use music as an effective motivational tool. You can choose your music based on your personal tastes, mood, or a specific situation and activity. The key is to choose music that helps you get motivated and stay motivated to take the right actions and perform at your peak.

Fans

Praise is an inexpensive motivational method. The genuine recognition and acknowledgement of an outstanding achievement is a powerful and proven form of extrinsic motivation. Too many people fail to understand and use the power of supportive people as a fitness motivation resource.

Fans are those people in your life that "have your back" and will always be rooting for you to win and succeed. They can be family members, friends, mentors, teammates, teachers, students, colleagues, coaches, or like-minded strangers.

The best ("core") fans are totally committed in their support and desire to see you succeed at fitness and weight loss. They will be there during the difficult times when your fitness motivation needs a charge. Treat these fans like invaluable treasures—because they are!

Family

There is nothing like having a supportive spouse, parent, child, best friend, or other close family member to help motivate you and keep you striving for improved fitness and health. These are essentially your *super fans*.

Sometimes, family members and friends can be *de-motivating*. Often, some people may not understand your fitness desires or challenges—and they may express this lack of understanding in the form of unproductive comments or suggestions.

In these instances, just ignore the unsupportive inputs--and choose to discuss your significant fitness and weight loss goals only with those who provide productive guidance and motivation. Be sure to express consistent thanks and gratitude to those who are your most ardent supporters.

Trainers and Coaches

I have not met a top athlete who did not credit a trainer or conditioning coach with having a significant impact on their personal fitness and athletic success. Quality trainers and coaches are invaluable to anyone who wants to achieve peak fitness levels.

A qualified fitness trainer can provide crucial knowledge and technical guidance on how to exercise and eat more effectively. Also, a trainer or coach can help you increase and sustain your fitness motivation.

Role Models

I have always been fascinated with the mental qualities and success strategies that differentiate ultra-high achievers from average achievers in fitness and sports.

Studying, interviewing, and modeling winners at the highest level is one of my personal motivation methods. I will typically focus on one role model at a time. Once I have integrated and started applying the key learnings from one high achiever, I will seek out another high-level fitness role model. It is a continuous process.

By studying those who have succeeded in losing weight and getting more fit, you will gain knowledge and insights that will help you achieve your fitness goals.

Pictures

You've probably heard the saying "a picture is worth a thousand words." As it relates to the development of your fitness motivation skills, the right pictures can be a great source of ongoing inspiration.

I've seen athletes make poster boards of a championship trophy and hang it in their rooms as a way to stay focused and motivated until they obtained the real thing.

You may choose to hang or download pictures of yourself when you were in the best physical shape of your life. Also, you may choose to use pictures of role models as a way to motivate yourself to get into better physical shape.

Conversely, you can use "before" pictures of your "out-of-shape" self as a way to stay motivated and moving toward your fitness and weight loss goals.

Visualization

Visualization is an internal picture—or a picture in your mind. Because visualization allows you to alter pictures instantly and completely, it is a powerful *and convenient* motivation tool.

I find that visualization works best when you use a *dual action technique*. First, you start by picturing yourself doing the activity or actions that lead to your fitness or weight loss goal. Second, you picture the actual moment or representation of success in achieving the goal.

For example, if your goal is to lose twenty pounds—you would first visualize yourself eating right and exercising regularly. Secondly, you would visualize yourself after you have achieved the weight loss. The second picture may consist of imagining yourself stepping on a scale that displays your target weight. Or, you may imagine your new body features and how attractive they are to others who are complimenting you on your improved appearance.

Self-Talk

Self-talk (done correctly) is a very effective programming and motivation tool. With productive and precise self-talk, you can provide instant and sustainable motivation. I suggest you get creative and find the right motivational sayings to help you start and stay in action. For example, I have used the following: "Let's do it!" "Let's get fit!" "I'm ready!" "I will do this!"

The key to effective self-motivation through self-talk is to use your body and emotions to generate increased energy and stronger positive connections with the success activity (such as exercise or healthy eating). You must "say it like you mean it!"

Self-talk works best when you say your motivational commands aloud. However, if you are not comfortable or able to do this--you may choose to use silent self-talk commands within your mind.

Use self-talk before every workout, exercise session, and meal to condition your mind to enter the "MotivateFit zone." You will find that your go-to motivational commands will eventually become automatic triggers that you can use to motivate yourself anytime.

Kinesiology

As a MotivateFit student, you need to have solutions for getting motivated and moving, even when you are not feeling up to it.

Kinesiology is the scientific study of human movement. One effective solution for overcoming inertia (or lack of motivation) is *movement*.

It is much easier to get motivated and stay motivated when you are in motion. If you will simply "get moving" and take that first action step—and the next step—you will become increasingly more motivated.

For example, if don't feel like exercising—simply put on your exercise clothes as the first action step and "just keep moving" (one simple simple step at a time). Before you know it, you will have completed another successful workout!

Social Circle

As humans, we are naturally susceptible to peer pressure. As a fitness motivation student, you can use this scientific fact to your advantage by associating with people who will strengthen and consistently renew your motivation to get fit and lose weight.

The people you surround yourself with either lift you up (and toward your fitness goals) or pull you down (and away from your fitness goals); they motivate you or drain you; they support you or criticize you; they make you cheerful or make you gloomy.

If someone regularly associates with underachievers, they may not become a total loser— but they will decrease their odds of achieving significant success and reaching their full potential. If you want to become a fitness and weight loss winner—*associate with winners!*

Declaration

A declaration is an explicit and formal statement or announcement. It is a public commitment. By "going public" with your fitness and weight loss goals, you can leverage the peer pressure factor to help initiate and maintain motivation.

You can declare your goals to your immediate family—or you can broaden the reach and motivational force of your declaration by proclaiming your goals to a wider circle of friends, colleagues, or team members.

Chapter 6

Willpower for Fitness and Weight Loss

Many people believe they could improve their lives if only they had more of that mysterious thing called willpower. With more self-control, we would all eat healthier, exercise regularly, save more for retirement, stop procrastinating, and achieve all sorts of positive goals.

According to the American Psychological Association--*not having willpower was the number one reason people cited for being unable to reach their goals and make successful lifestyle changes* related to their health and finances.

A growing body of evidence indicates that willpower and self-control are essential for a happy and healthy life. As a fitness motivation student, you must learn how to develop and maximize willpower and self-control, so that you can resist negative influences and eliminate bad habits that undermine your fitness and weight management.

We have many common names for willpower: self-control, impulse control, delayed gratification, resolve, or determination. According to most psychological scientists, willpower can be described as follows:

> * The ability to delay gratification, resisting short-term temptations in order to achieve long-term goals.
>
> * The capacity to override an unwanted or negative thought, feeling or impulse.
>
> * The ability to employ a "rational" cognitive system of behavior rather than an "irrational" emotional system.
>
> * Conscious regulation of the self by the self.
>
> * A limited resource capable of being depleted.

Motivation (covered in the previous chapter) is about increasing *desire to do something* that moves you closer toward your goals. Whereas, willpower is more about having the skills and ability to *resist or not do something* that conflicts with and undermines progress toward your goals.

The Science of Willpower

Two main areas of the brain contribute to the process of willpower--the limbic system (located right under the brain) and the prefrontal cortex (the front section of the brain right behind your forehead). These sections of the brain are linked closely together, and their communication efficiency determines how well you can exhibit willpower and self-control.

The limbic system is the "emotional" part of the brain. It is associated with your desires and urges for instant gratification. The prefrontal cortex is the "logical" part of the brain, which is associated with the cognitive function of rational thought, decision-making, and behavior regulation.

Whenever an emotional response is generated by the limbic system, the prefrontal cortex then interprets the response. This allows the prefrontal cortex to produce a logical behavioral response based on the situation. The more active your prefrontal cortex is--the greater your capacity for willpower and emotional control.

The willpower process is activated in response to an internal conflict. Let's use lunchtime as an example. The desire for instant gratification may cause an individual to order a supersized fast food lunch, followed by a cigarette break. Conversely, motivation and a stronger desire to exercise willpower may cause an individual to order a healthy and hearty salad, followed by a short walk.

One of the most consistent scientific findings about willpower is that it seems to be finite—that is, we only have so much during a 24-hour period and it runs out as we use it—and we need to replenish it regularly. *Willpower depends on the body's natural energy cycle and tends to be strongest at the beginning of the day.*

Trying to control your instant gratification desires, negative emotions, non-vital distractions, or simply refusing an unhealthy desert all tap the same source of mental strength known as willpower. The more we use willpower, the weaker it tends to get throughout the day.

Willpower is essentially like a muscle—it can be exhausted by overuse, but just like our physical muscles--*researchers believe we can strengthen our willpower and expand its capacity by training it.* Because willpower is like a muscle--you have to exhaust it in the short-term in order to build its strength in the long-term.

Your willpower is strengthened by doing anything that gets your brain out of its comfort zone in a healthy manner. When you actively work to develop your fitness motivation and health habits, you deplete your willpower in the process--but over time, the strength of your willpower increases--making you better able to demonstrate fitness motivation consistency for achieving your goals in the future.

The best part about creating a new willpower habit is that not only does it strengthen your MotivateFit skills--it also frees up more of your willpower for other things. When a decision evolves into a habit--it draws little, if any, energy from your willpower supply. The more healthy decisions and actions you can make habitual, the less impact and drain on your willpower you'll experience throughout the day.

This is why MotivateFit students with stronger self-control actually spend *less* time resisting desires than those with weaker self-control. By developing willpower, fitness motivation, and good habits— MotivateFit students can minimize the number of temptations they face by making daily fitness decisions and actions automatic.

The Marshmallow Experiment

The most persuasive evidence on willpower and delayed gratification comes from two studies that measured young children's self-control, and then kept track of them as they grew into adults.

The most well-known experiment, the "marshmallow experiment," was started in the 1960s by psychologist Walter Mischel. He offered four-year-olds the choice of a marshmallow now, or two if they could wait fifteen minutes. He and other researchers then tracked the performance of these children, as they became adults. They found that children who resisted temptation ("high delayers") achieved greater academic success, better health, and lower rates of marital separation and divorce. Mischel concluded that the ability to delay gratification constituted "*a protective buffer against the development of all kinds of vulnerabilities later in life.*"

In a second study, 1,000 children were tracked from birth to the age of thirty-two. The researchers found that childhood self-control predicted physical health, substance dependence, personal finances, and criminal offenses. This was true even when other factors such as intelligence and social class were considered. The researchers even compared sibling pairs and found that the sibling in each pair with lower measured willpower or self-control had more negative life outcomes, despite shared family background.

Below is a link to a Marshmallow experiment video:

http://goo.gl/h3dA6d

The Marshmallow experiment provides evidence on the lifelong impact of being conditioned to exercise willpower vs. succumb to instant gratification.

MotivateFit students know that willpower is a core component and skill of all highly fit individuals. Increased willpower will directly increase fitness motivation, exercise consistency, and healthy eating.

The Willpower Journey

In order to increase your willpower, you must learn to enjoy the moments and process of exercising and strengthening your willpower. This attitude and approach to willpower development will help you reach your fitness goals faster and maintain your success longer.

If you are going to be a highly fit individual for life--you must fall in love with the destination (goal), *and* you must fall in love with traveling the actual journey (which is the process of developing willpower and other fitness motivation skills).

Use the pleasure of seeing yourself growing and developing unstoppable willpower as added motivation to continue exercising your willpower until it becomes automatic. When I was first learning how to strengthen my willpower, I would pat myself on the back (literally) and say "great job" every time I exercised willpower throughout the day.

I suggest you use this simple reinforcing tool. You can insert your name to make it feel even more personal. And, don't worry if you are reluctant about shouting to yourself in a crowded room. You can pat yourself on the back and silently tell yourself that you did a "great job" whenever you exercise willpower.

You can also use the *pain* of potentially seeing yourself fall short of maximizing your potential as motivation to exercise regular willpower and ensure significant progress toward your goals.

Do not fall victim to the bad advice that you should reward yourself (associate pleasure) with the very things that you will use willpower to avoid or stop doing. The problem with this bad advice—for example, having a piece of chocolate cake to reward yourself for losing three pounds this week—is that it undermines the development and optimization of your willpower and fitness motivation habits.

Inevitably, you will experience lapses as you are developing your willpower and self-control skills. But, please make the following promise to yourself: *Never* say—"oh well forget it" or allow yourself to spiral out of control just because you lose one episode of "willpower vs. instant gratification."

MotivateFit students—and even world-class athletes--have occasional lapses in willpower. The difference between MotivateFit students (or professional athletes) and the average person is that their willpower lapses are much less frequent (perhaps once every month or maybe once every week—as opposed to once every day or even once every hour for those with nonexistent willpower).

MotivateFit students typically have willpower lapses on things that are not critical to their key goals. Whereas, those with low self-control skills will experience consistent willpower lapses on important decisions and actions related to their key goals.

Conserving Your Willpower

Because willpower is a real, finite energy, the question that naturally arises is; how can you conserve and strengthen this force to maximize your fitness motivation skills?

How do you generate enough willpower energy to strive towards and achieve success? The first step is to *consciously conserve* this energy, by keeping it from being squandered--and saving it for the fitness and weight loss goals that are most important and impactful to you.

Following are seven specific and proven ways to help conserve your willpower energy.

1. Clarify and prioritize goals

2. Plan and prepare

3. Simplify your life

4. Get enough sleep

5. Maintain general health

6. Track results

7. Eliminate willpower killers

Let's review and discuss the seven willpower conservation solutions.

Clarify and Prioritize Goals

My personal experience with clients and athletes, has taught me that *limiting your focus to one or two significant fitness goals at a time will dramatically improve your odds of success.*

Because willpower is a finite resource—chasing too many goals at once will drain your mental strength, and will not provide sufficient willpower for any of your goals. The result is typically failure in most, if not all of your goals. Instead, you should funnel your willpower towards one or two key fitness goals at any given time.

Clear goals provide clear focus for your brain and added motivation to exercise your willpower. If you set S.M.A.R.T. (specific, measurable, actionable, realistic, and timed) goals—you will be ten times more likely to reach your goals than those who have poorly articulated or "non-smart" goals.

Plan and Prepare

Science and daily life have both provided ample evidence that *planners are winners*. This is why I've incorporated this crucial element into the MotivateFit Method.

You cannot achieve sustainable success of any significant measure without learning how to properly plan and prepare. Plans don't need to be complicated. Often, it's the simplest plans that are most effective.

The definition of *luck is when preparation meets opportunity*. If you learn to appreciate, enjoy, and invest in planning and preparation--you will excel in fitness, weight management, and all areas of your life.

Simplify Your Life

Simplicity is a constant and trustworthy companion for all peak performers in life. Simplification leads to less clutter in your mind, which helps to conserve your valuable willpower.

Following are some recommendations to help you simplify your life and mind to better support your fitness and weight loss goals.

Automate Routine Tasks

Whenever you recognize a specific and necessary decision or activity that demands repetition—begin to seek out ways to automate the task. This will free up time and mental energy. The best way make a task more efficient varies, but options include--technology solutions; improved processes; and delegation or outsourcing.

You should evaluate any repetitive task occasionally and ask yourself if it is necessary. If a task is simply not necessary, eliminate it.

Use To-Do Lists

Lists are a very effective way to save time and free up your mind power for more critical tasks. Using lists will improve your productivity and effectiveness. Every successful individual has learned how to use lists to help manage performance and deliver superior results.

You can choose to keep important lists (such as a healthy diet grocery list) in your smartphone, or you can simply use pen and paper.

Get Organized

Highly successful and fit people place a high value on their time. A commitment to becoming and staying organized will save time and reduce stress, which makes it easier to use your willpower for fitness and weight loss.

Chronic disorganization will deplete your willpower. Simplify your life and protect your mental energy by implementing simple routines to stay organized at home, work, school, and during travel.

Get Enough Sleep and Rest

The most successful athletes and MotivateFit students make time for adequate sleep and rest. Being well-rested will have a positive impact on your fitness motivation and physical performance.

Following are a few outcomes from scientific sleep studies conducted on athletes:

*Sleep improves split-second decision-making ability by 4.3%.

*Tennis players get a 42% boost in hitting accuracy when they get adequate sleep.

*An athlete's maximum bench press drops by 20 pounds after four days of inadequate sleep.

Similar outcomes related to sleeping habits were found when observing and testing business executives. The more rested they were, the better they performed on cognitive skill tests and decision-making assessments.

Sleep

Sleep is a natural periodic state of unconscious rest for the mind and body. Adequate sleep is vital to willpower functioning, fitness motivation, and sports performance.

Research suggests that even small amounts of sleep deprivation will take a significant toll on your health, mood, cognitive capacity, and productivity. *Conserving, exercising, and managing willpower becomes exponentially harder as sleep deprivation increases.*

Don't fool yourself by bragging to your colleagues and friends about how you can function on a few hours of sleep per night! Champion athletes and highly fit individuals understand the importance and power of this most basic human function. Sleep is much more important than your ego!

LeBron James is one of the most celebrated and gifted professional athletes in professional sports today. In addition to innate talent and dedicated training—LeBron credits healthy sleeping habits as one of the keys to his peak performance consistency.

During particularly intense periods, such as during the playoffs--LeBron often sleeps up to 12 hours a day. This may seem like a lot for most people, but elite athletes place an enormous amount of stress on their bodies and minds—which requires significant sleep time for complete repair and recuperation.

As a MotivateFit student—you should get adequate sleep each night if you want to conserve your willpower and keep your fitness motivation functioning at a high level.

Naps are a natural and powerful willpower conservation tool that you can use when you don't have a lot of time for regular sleep--or simply need a boost in physical or mental energy. Short, effective naps can be as little as five minutes--and longer, more restorative naps can be as long as ninety minutes.

Maintain General Health

For most elite athletes—exercise is part of their job. For anyone outside of sports—consistent exercise and healthy eating have been linked to increased willpower. In essence, willpower improves your fitness—and as your fitness improves, you will gain increased willpower. It's a really nice "circle of success!"

Certainly, you will be better equipped to conserve and exercise willpower if you are effectively managing your stress and mood. Recent studies have shown that exercise is effective in reducing stress and even short-term bouts of depression.

Suffering from a known or unknown physical or mental ailment can have an adverse effect on your willpower and fitness motivation.   I recommend scheduling regular physical exams with a medical doctor. You should view your doctor as a key member of your fitness motivation success team.

Track Results

Remember, our goal is to make sure you get the highest return on your investment of willpower each day by applying your limited mind energy to your top one or two fitness goals. This ensures that you will get better results and make faster progress.

You can reach your fitness and weight loss goals more quickly if you take the time to evaluate your performance and results on a regular basis. Using this proven strategy--you will always know what's working and what's not working to help you exercise and eat right more consistently.

By knowing the key drivers of your success— you can focus your willpower on those decisions and activities that are proving to be most beneficial.

Eliminate Willpower Killers

Drain people

People who pull you toward negative instant gratification decisions or activities that directly conflict with your fitness and weight loss goals are drain people.

Don't tax your willpower unnecessarily. Eliminate or avoid drain people as much as possible.

When you can't avoid drain people, seek to minimize their impact by making your goals clear and willpower evident. Typically, drain people want to hang out with like-minded people and don't want to be reminded of their own shortcomings or lack of fitness motivation.

Burnout

Remember, you only have so much willpower available in a 24-hour period before your willpower starts to wane and become more difficult to maintain due to declining energy or sleepiness.

Be careful of overworking and overtraining because it can lead to burnout. Symptoms of burnout include a noticeable decline in motivation, willpower, performance, and results. Adhering to this warning and avoiding burnout is typically difficult for uninformed "Type A" personalities and perfectionists who want to apply willpower to every task throughout the entire day.

Remember—for the best long-term results, you should conserve your willpower for daily decisions and activities that will directly impact your crucial fitness goals. Don't waste precious willpower energy on insignificant goals. As author Richard

Carlson exulted in his bestselling book—"D*on't Sweat The Small Stuff.*"

Drugs and Alcohol

Fact: Drugs, medications, and alcohol can impair mental capacity and weaken your willpower. If you want to conserve willpower and fitness motivation, do not ingest or abuse mind-altering substances.

Strengthening Your Willpower and Self-Control

If you want to increase your ability to exercise more willpower and self-control—you must consciously train and develop this mental skill. While there are many ways to *conserve* your willpower, there is really just one way to strengthen it--by *consciously* working toward a goal or habit that exercises (challenges) your self-control.

Remember, developing willpower and self-control requires that you condition yourself to push past the initial pull of instinctive emotional responses. You must learn to quickly override negative thoughts and feelings that might lead to unproductive decisions and actions.

The following is a simple process that has proven itself very effective in helping MotivateFit students improve their willpower skills.

3-Step Willpower Activation Process

The process of consciously activating your willpower involves the following three steps:

1. **Pause**

2. **Erase**

3. **Replace**

Pause

Before making a decision or taking any action, you must learn to *instantly engage your conscious mind* and refuse to let emotions drive you toward unproductive instant gratification.

When faced with a desire to act or decide on an unproductive impulse, the first thing you must condition yourself to do is simply *pause!*

Stop! Take a slow deep breath. Relax your body and mind. This literally takes only two to five seconds.

The objective of this *power pause* is to quickly reduce the intensity of the unproductive temptation. In addition, this step is designed to give you instant physical control.

Erase

Once you have gained physical control, your immediate next step is to *erase* the unproductive thought, distraction, or temptation. You must (visually and verbally) erase the threat to your willpower with deliberate and confident force!

You can imagine the thought disappearing— or, you can silently shout "NO" to the negative temptation while erasing it from your mind. This takes one to two seconds.

Focus on becoming faster and faster when practicing erasing. As you become more conditioned—you will find that you can erase potential distractions within a split-second.

Replace

The final step in gaining control over unproductive thoughts and feelings is to *activate your willpower.*

Because you have taken instant control of your body and mind—and eliminated the unproductive willpower threat--you will now *replace the unproductive thought with a productive thought,* such as your fitness or weight loss goal. This final step will direct your powerful willpower muscles to make the right decision and take productive action!

Be sure to direct all of your positive mental and emotional focus to your most relevant fitness

goal. This takes five to ten seconds. You can use visual imagery, self-talk, or productive action to reinforce the fact that *your willpower and fitness goals will win when confronted with unproductive thoughts, temptations, and distractions.*

The *replace* step is critical because it validates your personal power and represents the precise point of willpower strengthening within the brain.

The motivating strength of your fitness and weight loss goals, coupled with the use of this simple process will maximize your willpower and remove obstacles to daily effectiveness.

I guarantee that if you practice this simple 3-step process consistently, you will start to feel and see a difference in your willpower very quickly. Within a few days or weeks, you will notice that you can instantly apply the willpower activation process in real-time situations without even thinking about it.

Willpower and Self-Control Exercises

The following are specific exercises to help strengthen your willpower for fitness and weight loss. You can use the 3-step willpower activation process when practicing these self-control exercises.

In addition to using the exercises within this book--I encourage you to be creative and come up with your own unique and customized ways to challenge and grow your self-control skills.

Daily Jumpstart

Exercise your willpower by resisting the urge to snooze or stay in bed upon arising first thing in the morning. As soon as the alarm goes off, or you naturally wake up—immediately get up out of the bed! You can then yawn, stretch, take a few deep breaths, repeat your key fitness goals a few times (programming), and ease into your morning routine, which should include exercise or a healthy breakfast.

Deliberate Delay

Practicing the "art of denial" is an effective way to exercise your willpower. The focal point of your delay should be something that you value and view as a motivating reward.

The following are a few examples of deliberate delays.

*Food – Consciously wait a few seconds before eating your first or last bite of food so that you can really gauge your hunger. Delay going back for more food or a second plate until you have waited at least fifteen to twenty minutes, which is the time it takes your brain to communicate to your stomach that you may be full.

*Entertainment – Delay before you instinctively reach for your smartphone every thirty seconds. Delay before you rush to read emails or social media posts. Delay before you turn on the TV and grab a snack when you arrive at home.

*Travel – Use your willpower to delay the instinct to call and chat with a family member or friend while driving home. Delay turning on your car radio (if this is your usual pattern). Instead, try to drive along with thoughts of your key fitness goals for a few minutes before turning on the radio.

Distraction Denial

I have found this simple exercise to be very powerful in keeping my willpower muscles tuned up and ready for the bigger, more significant challenges to self-control.

For the distraction denial exercise, you can use any smaller decisions throughout your day to challenge and strengthen your willpower.

For example, let's assume that you are in the middle of preparing dinner—but you have to stop for a bathroom break. On your way back to the kitchen, you walk pass something that is untidy or out of place and you instinctively want to pick it up or put it back in place (perhaps clothing, or a kid's toy, or a household item).

Another example--you have a thought about someone you want to call--or a small task comes to mind that needs to be completed.

Instead of giving in to the impulse—choose to exercise your willpower and go right back to the preparation of your delicious and nutritious dinner. It's not that the potential distraction would have undermined your ultimate and ongoing success—but it's a great opportunity for you to "flex" your willpower muscles in a quick and easy way by saying "no" to distractions. It reinforces the belief and fact that *you are in control of your decisions and actions.*

Immediate Action

Learn to exercise your willpower by replacing thoughts with immediate action. When you know you should do something right now, and you really do have the time—just do it now!

* You just arrived at home after a long, brutal day at work. You want to hit the couch and grab the remote control to your TV—even though you planned to exercise upon arriving at home. Go exercise. Just do it now!

*You just finished eating a very enjoyable dinner at home. You don't feel like washing the dishes before you turn on the TV. Wash the dishes. Just do it now!

*You know that you should use part of your lunch hour to register for that leadership course or make that important networking call to an important contact. Just do it now!

*You are single and not sure if the attractive single person you're chatting with at the fundraiser event will go out on a date with you. Simply ask. Just do it now!

Priority Push

Stop putting low impact tasks before high impact tasks. They are not equal. This pattern sabotages progress and success. Manage your time more effectively and maximize your willpower usage by working on higher priority tasks related to your fitness and weight loss before investing time in lower priority tasks.

Review your schedule and to-do list daily. Make sure you are prioritizing fitness related tasks (such as exercise) that will have the most impact on moving you toward significant health.

Chapter 7

Improve Your Diet

The Sustainable Fitness Diet

If you want to maintain motivation for fitness and weight loss—it is important for you to make a shift in your perception of what diet really means.

The word "diet" is not an evil four-letter word. It is a good thing with a questionable perception. Most people have attached overwhelming negativity to the word. In order to succeed where you may have failed before, you must remove all of the twenty-first century hype and get "back to the basics."

Most people mistakenly equate the word diet with the reduction of caloric intake for the purpose of weight loss. Be honest. When you think of diet, you probably think of eating small amounts of less than tasty foods and fighting off hunger and cravings while you're doing it!

Despite the perceptions and false claims perpetuated by the weight loss industry and the constant flow of "miracle" diets and pills—a diet (at its root) is simply *the regular intake of food and drink consumed for nourishment.*

Every human being is on a diet. Obesity and the flip side, malnutrition, both result from an **imbalanced** diet.

As a MotivateFit student—your goal is to achieve a balanced and healthy diet that promotes the proper energy balance for your specific body, activity levels, and fitness goals.

Isn't it time you let go of the "deprivation mentality" and *make the conscious shift from temporary diet pain to permanent diet pleasure.*

You can start this psychological transformation in thinking by affirming your commitment to the fitness lifestyle, which requires that you provide your body with the nourishment necessary to perform at your best every day.

As children, we automatically ate whatever our parents placed before us because our food decisions were made for us. We were not responsible for them, or held accountable. We merely made judgments based upon taste. We liked macaroni and cheese; we didn't like broccoli or brussel sprouts. Most people continue this programmed behavior into adulthood.

As an adult, it is now your responsibility (and within your power) to develop a better relationship with food based on love, nourishment, and respect-- for the gift of your body and for the gift of healthy food, which fuels your daily life and fitness success.

Your body consists of many biological and physiological functions that support life. It requires nutrients, minerals, and other supportive elements. It relies upon you to provide those elements in a balanced manner. Any excess or deficit has an accumulated effect on the body.

Age and genetics notwithstanding--your current body and physical capabilities are primarily the result of your behavior, decisions, and actions over time. Each time you sit down to eat, you can *choose to reward your body with a healthy and balanced meal—* which will result in increased energy, fitness, and beauty.

Choosing a healthy diet does not mean that you have to forsake taste. Taste is not to be ignored. You are allowed to eat those things that have the flavors you personally prefer. The key is to choose those items that have the tastes you like and provide the proper fuel your body needs.

With your MotivateFit skills—*you can make the shift from feasting to fueling*. MotivateFit students view all food as fuel and energy for their precious bodies. Failures in fitness and weight loss view food as entertainment; or a punishment; or a reward; or a stress reducer. If any of these describes your relationship with food—you can change this and develop a healthier, more practical, and beneficial relationship with food that supports your stated fitness goals.

Food is not a therapist--or entertainer--or disciplinarian! Most people overcomplicate the concept of dieting. You can enjoy the experience of eating, and savoring flavors and taste, while fueling your body and not feasting to overfill.

The key is to keep your diet simple and healthy. Just view a healthy diet as one in which food is fuel and you have the choice of what kind and how much fuel you use to power your body.

Always think healthy, balanced, satisfying, and sustainable when making diet choices.

Don't expect to find the perfect solution off-the-shelf diet. There is no such thing. The best diet for you is one that you develop and customize over time based on sound nutritional science, your fitness goals, your energy requirements, and your taste preferences.

Allow yourself sufficient time to develop effective and healthy eating patterns and habits. *It takes time to develop a healthy and sustainable diet.* Let results be your ultimate guide. If you are losing the desired weight, feeling more energetic, and are able to sustain for the long-term—your diet and eating habits are working. This is the sustainable diet for a fitness lifestyle!

Balance F.A.T. in Your Diet

F.A.T. stands for *frequency, amount,* and *type.* F.A.T. balance is the active management of frequency, amount, and type as it relates to your sustainable fitness diet. More specifically, it involves the following:

*Frequency of food intake.

*Amount of food intake.

*Type of food intake.

F.A.T. balancing provides you with a concept and tool that, when applied to your daily diet, will allow you to more easily achieve and maintain your weight loss and fitness. I've witnessed many clients who were able to maintain healthy eating patterns with less stress by using the F.A.T. balancing strategy when compared to more extreme, rigorous, or one-dimensional dieting plans.

Fuel Up Regularly

Frequency of food intake helps maintain the body's proper energy balance. Refueling regularly also helps control the amount of intake. When you eat frequently, you will naturally eat less at each sitting. You are better able to manage the amount you consume because you will never get too hungry.

Hunger is a sign that the body needs fuel—calories and nutrients—to keep running effectively. Avoid allowing yourself to get too hungry or too full. Try to maintain balance and simplicity. Eat when you are a little bit hungry (to help avoid binges)—and stop eating once you are comfortably full.

Do not eat until you are stuffed, or you are likely to trigger a guilt, starvation, binge cycle that disrupts your healthy eating patterns and compromises your fitness and weight loss goals.

Reject Portion Distortion

Amount of food intake is the greatest challenge to achieving and managing weight. For most people in developed countries--food is plentiful and affordable. We have embraced the concept of "supersizing" meals.

This vast abundance of food and increase in portion sizes is a major contributing factor for the 65% of Americans who are now overweight. The overweight and obesity epidemic is a crisis and health care issue that crosses all racial, gender, cultural, and age groups.

The solution is not to deny all of our favorite foods. It's not that you can't have a slice of pie, a piece of cake, potato chips, a soda, or even a crisp piece of fried chicken. But you should not have a *whole* pie, a *wedge* of cake, an entire *bucket* of chicken or a *gallon* of soda!

Portion is the amount of a specific food that you choose to eat, whenever you choose to eat it. Portions of food items in restaurants and grocery stores have grown increasingly larger. Today's one-person portion would have fed two people just twenty years ago.

As a MotivateFit student, you must pay close attention to portions and servings sizes. Always pause to think about calorie content and the number of servings (amount) you are actually going to consume based on your body's true energy demands.

Enjoy a Variety of Foods

Type of food intake is the third component of F.A.T. Balancing. The types of foods you choose will play a major role in achieving the fitness and weight loss you desire.

There is a great deal of information regarding healthier foods versus less healthy foods. There are simple, basic things to keep in mind. The goal is to consciously improve the health quotient of your food selections over time until you develop the habit of making healthier food choices automatic.

Try to include a wide variety of nutrient dense foods in your diet. *Nutrient-dense foods are those that provide substantial amounts of vitamins and minerals, and relatively few calories.*

Avoid any diets that restrict any food groups or key nutrients. Include all food groups in your diet, because each group provides a wide array of nutrients in substantial amounts. Vegetables, complex carbs, fruits, lean proteins, whole grains, and healthy fats such as mono-unsaturated and poly-unsaturated fats, should be emphasized, as they satisfy the body longer and more completely.

Nutrient-dense versions of foods provide a way to meet nutrition needs while avoiding the over-consumption of calories and of food components such as trans fats and saturated fats. For easier weight and fitness maintenance—you should minimize simple sugars, saturated and trans-fats, cholesterol, salt, and alcohol.

Low-nutrient-dense foods supply calories but have very few or no nutrients. As a result, you will still have cravings and overeat. The greater the consumption of foods or beverages that are low-nutrient dense, the more difficult it is to consume enough nutrients without gaining weight.

Foods that are low-nutrient dense have "empty calories." Empty calorie foods have a lot of calories and no nutritional value. By merely cutting empty calories, you can lose weight. Substitute zero calorie drinks for sugary sodas. Increase water intake and substitute fruit for fruit juices when possible.

As you reduce low-nutrient-dense foods in exchange for nutrient-dense foods in your diet, you will increase your energy level and reduce your hunger level.

It is critical to respect special dietary needs for pregnant women, seniors, diabetics, and those with certain diseases or food allergies. Before declaring yourself allergic to any food ingredients, such as gluten, I recommend seeking out a board certified allergist for food allergy testing.

Dining Out

Making healthy food choices when eating out can be challenging. Many restaurants and fast food chains have made strides to offer health and diet-friendly options—as well as transparency in calories. Be vigilant when ordering. Pay attention to the menu descriptions so that you can choose healthier alternatives.

High-fat restaurant selections are described as: Alfredo, au gratin, batter dipped béarnaise, escalloped, breaded, creamy, crispy, flaky, fried, hollandaise, puffed, sautéed, and tempura. Low-fat restaurant selections are: baked, smoked, flame-cooked, broiled, steamed, poached, roasted, marinara, and grilled.

Below are additional tips on eating healthy while dining out.

Appetizers: Choose fresh fruits and vegetables without sauces, broth-based soups, and salads with low-fat or fat-free salad dressing on the side, avoiding croutons, heavy cheese, and avocado.

Beverages: Ice water, club soda, zero-calorie sodas, and coffee or tea without cream or sugar. Limit alcoholic beverages.

Sandwiches: Order lower-calorie fillings such as lean beef, chicken, turkey, and tuna, unless high in mayonnaise or other oil. Use mustard, lettuce, and tomato, while ordering spreads to be served separately.

Specialty Restaurants—Asian, Mexican, Italian, Indian, and Greek: Avoid deep-fried and battered fried selections, fried rice, sauces and gravies, cream and butter sauces, sour cream, large amounts of cheese, and clarified butter (ghee). Try stir-fried, grilled, or steamed.

Fast Food: Order a small hamburger without cheese, plain baked potato, grilled chicken sandwich, roast beef sandwich without sauce or cheese, baked fish, taco, or fajita.

Salad Bar: Select raw vegetables with reduced-calorie or fat-free dressing, chick peas, cottage cheese, diced ham, marinated beets and mushrooms, fresh fruit, or bean salad. Beware of high-calorie salad bar items. Substitute vinegar or lemon juice as dressing.

Cafeteria: Yogurt, chili and raw green salads with reduced or fat-free dressings are good options. Many cafeterias are increasing their healthy food selections.

Breakfast Bar or Restaurant: Keeping in mind serving size, choose eggs or egg whites, whole grain cereal, oatmeal, yogurt, fresh fruit, or 100% fruit juice. Choose smaller portion sizes if you select waffles, pancakes, or french toast—and consider using no butter or low-calorie syrup. Avoid the mammoth muffins.

Vending Machine: For a quick boost, choose trail mix, dried fruit mix, peanut butter crackers, fig bars, 100% fruit juice, or pretzels.

Mall: Look for the healthier choices. Pick a soft pretzel without cheese, frozen yogurt, vegetable pizza slice, and plain popcorn or tostada chips with salsa.

Deli: Select wisely. Review the menu nutrition information. Choose whole wheat bread, turkey breast, smoked turkey, ham or roast beef, grilled chicken salad, vegetable soup, or vinegar-based coleslaw.

Shopping for Food

Avoid spur-of-the-moment grocery shopping. Make a detailed list that includes lower-calorie, healthier choices, and never shop when you are hungry. If possible, take the time to read the nutrition labels so that you can make healthier selections.

Nutritional Supplements

Many MotivateFit students use nutritional supplements to help maintain their basic physical and mental health. Despite the best intentions to eat a well-balanced diet every day, the vast majority of people will fall short. At a minimum, nutritional supplements offer insurance against nutritional deficiency. Optimally, nutritional supplements can improve function and performance.

Ideally, you should take a vitamin deficiency test to see which vitamins are lacking in your daily diet. You can then take the vitamins you need to make up for the deficiency. This test will also prevent you from spending money on supplements you don't need.

Search online for a local and licensed nutritionist. If you cannot locate a nutritionist, ask your personal physician if they can test you, or refer you to someone who can.

I will avoid recommending a particular brand of vitamins. I will just say that a good multivitamin that includes all of the necessary daily nutrients is a good start. You can try additional products to see if they enhance your health and fitness, but you should consult your physician.

Because nutritional supplements can be expensive and sometimes dangerous, you should be wary of outlandish or unproven claims about benefits and results. If you have questions about a supplement, talk to a qualified health care professional.

Chapter 8

Increase Your Physical Activity

Physical activity is an essential key to lasting fitness and weight loss. And, of course—getting and staying motivated to be active is the fuel for a fitness lifestyle.

Physical activity involves any body movement produced by skeletal muscles and resulting in expenditure of energy. Exercise is a subset of physical activity that is planned and structured, with repetitive movement. Its main objective is to improve or maintain physical fitness.

This targeted type of fitness activity may be aerobic, focusing on the cardio-respiratory functions--or strength training, focusing on muscular strength and endurance--or flexibility training that focuses on the range of motion of various body joints.

Exercise Science Simplified

Physical activities specifically designed to improve or maintain health and fitness are based upon the principles of overload or specificity. To have a positive effect upon one of the body's physiological systems, such as the cardio-respiratory system--the aerobic physical activity performed *must require* that system to work harder than it is used to working. This *overload* of the system, places a demand upon the body to respond at the increased or overload level.

The overload for strength improvement is different from that for aerobic improvement. For strength training, a muscle or muscle group is specifically targeted with a specific demand, and results in a specific response. This principle of human performance is called *specificity*.

When operating within the guidelines of safety and the relative ability to perform the physical activity (tolerance), the body will adapt and demonstrate improved performance.

Physical Activity and Fitness Motivation

Regular effective exercise is one of the best investments you can make in your body and mind. It helps prevent and control many diseases and ailments. Also, *regular effective exercise is the single greatest determinant of long-term weight loss success.*

The more you exercise regularly—the more motivated you will become to get fit and stay fit!

The breakdown of food and its transformation into energy is a function of the body's metabolism process. Positively affecting metabolism advances weight loss. As discussed previously, there are three elements that affect the metabolism process:

Resting Metabolic Rate: The amount of energy, measured in calories that supports essential body functions and daily tasks.

Thermic Effect of Food: The amount of energy from calories that supports digestion, absorption, and the metabolism of food.

Physical Activity: The greatest opportunity to impact the metabolic process is with physical activity. Physical activity improves metabolism in two ways. First, it *increases calories burned* by increasing activity through cardiovascular exercise. Secondly, physical activity *improves resting metabolic rate* through strength training, which supports the body's natural ability to burn more calories at the same given weight. In other words--*one pound of muscle burns more calories than one pound of fat.*

Achieving weight loss without exercise and physical activity is the main cause of weight cycling commonly called yo-yo dieting. The on again, off again nature of highly-restrictive dieting, without exercise and increased physical activity, means that you must repeat the low-calorie diet to maintain the achieved weight loss.

Failure to maintain the weight loss without increased physical activity is predictable. Diets that are too restrictive, or too low in calories can only be sustained short-term because of the effect on the body and its systems. Once the low-calorie diet is completed, the dieter is forced to further restrict food intake in order to maintain the weight loss achieved— which becomes physiologically and psychologically impossible over an extended period of time.

Because extreme dieters are not burning the additional calories through increased physical activity, their only option is to recycle the low-calorie diet after they eventually fail (and gain all of the weight back). This is not only emotionally and psychologically destructive, but over time, it is also physiologically damaging.

Extreme dieting will help you achieve initial weight loss. However, many scientific studies have consistently proven that exercise is the most critical link to successful weight management once you achieve your target weight.

Your goal as a MotivateFit student is to live a fitness lifestyle--not a yo-yo dieting lifestyle of continually recycled fad diets.

The combination of healthy diet and exercise as a means of increasing fitness motivation and achieving weight loss freedom has been tried, tested, and proven repeatedly in clinical studies. This is no fad or fantasy! A consistently healthy diet and regular exercise are, in fact, the real miracle solution!

Oops, the secret is out! But truthfully, it has been a secret hidden in plain sight. Note that this wording is on all fad diet and weight loss products: *"When used in conjunction with a healthy diet and exercise, product XYZ has been shown to reduce body fat."* No kidding!

Benefits of Exercise

The benefits of increased physical activity extend beyond fitness and weight management. Consistent exercise and physical activity will improve the quality of your life in many significant ways—both physically and psychologically.

Physical Benefits of Exercise

Attractive Appearance: Increased physical attractiveness will result from developing a more toned and sculpted body composition. When dieting, your body shrinks, but it will retain its shape, looking the same. Exercise, particularly strength training, actually allows you to sculpt your new "smaller" body, so that it is not only smaller, but more esthetically pleasing.

Improves Balance: The improved strength level resulting from physical activity will improve physical balance and coordination.

Energy Level: Consistent exercise promotes a greater level of endurance. You will experience fewer peaks and valleys of energy throughout the day. This reduces any dependence on stimulants. It also encourages a natural sleep without the use of drugs. You will be more restful and awake more refreshed.

Improves Sex Life: Increased energy level and a sculpted physique must count for something in the bedroom. What do you think? Enjoy!

Medical Benefits of Exercise

Heart: Daily physical activity can help prevent heart disease and stroke by strengthening your heart muscle, lowering your blood pressure, leveling out cholesterol levels, and improving blood flow. These same benefits extend to the lungs and all cardiorespiratory functions.

Non-Insulin Dependent (Type 2) Diabetes: By reducing body fat, physical activity can help prevent and control this type of diabetes.

Obesity: Physical activity helps to reduce body fat by building or preserving muscle mass and improving the body's ability to use calories.

Back Pain: Regular exercise helps to prevent back pain by encouraging strength and flexibility.

Osteoporosis: Regular weight-bearing or strength training exercises promote bone formation and may prevent many forms of bone loss associated with aging, especially for women.

Emotional Benefits of Exercise

Stress Management: Allows you to manage stress, reduce anxiety, and feel more in control of your life.

Self Esteem: Regular physical activity can improve your mood. Exercise has been shown to reduce symptoms of depression, while providing an encouraging sense of accomplishment.

Mental Benefits of Exercise

Regular physical activity and exercise can help ward off the deterioration of your mental skills as you age. Concentration, focus, memory, and overall improved performance are side-effects of being active.

The brain releases endorphins during some types of physical activity. They serve as the body's natural pain reliever and mood enhancer. This naturally-produced mood elevator is a motivating byproduct embraced by all MotivateFit students as a way to maintain their fitness motivation.

Boost Metabolism Naturally

As discussed earlier—the most effective and natural way to boost your metabolism is with physical activity. This can be accomplished using a variety of physical activities that provide specific benefits for the body and its physiological systems.

The *type* of exercise you choose will determine the best *frequency* and *amount* of exercise. If you choose lower intensity, or easier exercise options—you will be able to do them more frequently and for longer periods of time. On the other hand, if you prefer higher intensity exercise—you will have to engage in this type of exercise less frequently and/or for shorter periods of time in order to avoid injury and have sufficient time for your body to recover.

Important: *The most common cause of exercise dropout is overtraining or burnout. In order to increase and maintain your fitness motivation—you must actively avoid overtraining by choosing a type, frequency, and amount of exercise that is challenging but enjoyable for you.*

The MotivateFit method and philosophy strongly supports the "take it slow and consistent" approach to exercise and fitness motivation. Avoid pushing yourself too hard too fast. Your body and mind must be trained to adapt to regular exercise over time.

Also, progressive and consistent exercise must be balanced with sufficient recovery time. The harder you exercise—the more time your body and mind need to recover and recuperate.

Types of Exercise

The two types of exercise are *primary* and *supplemental.*

Primary Exercise

Primary exercises are natural daily physical activities. These are generally unstructured physical tasks performed during your daily life.

Primary exercises can include the following:

*Walking the dog

*Climbing stairs

*Lifting boxes

*Taking out the trash

*Cleaning the house

*Washing the car

*Playing physical games with children

*Gardening

*Window shopping at the mall

These and other similar activities are the way that most people get exercise in their daily lives. In centuries past, primary exercise was enough to effectively manage our weight, simply because we participated in more primary exercise activities.

Daily life in past centuries consisted of many acts of physical labor. Farming, working, cooking, washing, walking, shopping, cleaning, literally "running errands," and even using the bathroom meant a trip outside and around to the back of the house. There weren't super-sized meals, time and labor-saving devices, and sedentary jobs and lifestyles.

In this modern age, you could spend twenty-four hours in a 500 square foot high-rise apartment going from the bed, bathroom, microwave in the kitchen, television in front of the sofa, laptop on the end table, and receiving all the latest news and information from around the world--all before settling in to listen to your iPod. In that twenty-four hour period, you may not even have walked a total of one hundred yards! However, you probably ate much more than you needed to provide the calories you used for fuel to carry out the physical activities of your day.

Supplemental Exercise

The regularity of not balancing our activity level with our calorie consumption has resulted in many of us being unfit and overweight. In many cases today, we simply don't get enough primary exercise.

For this modern world, expanding the physical activities in our lives to include **supplemental exercise** addresses the need for increased activity--to overcome a sedentary lifestyle due to technological conveniences--and an increased calorie intake due to an abundance of faster, cheaper foods.

Supplemental exercise is a great tool for getting fit and accelerating weight loss. Also, supplemental exercise can help you overcome "plateaus" and sticking points that you may experience with dieting alone.

Primary exercise is a great starting point for totally sedentary individuals. However, if you want to maximize your fitness motivation and physical transformation—you should engage in regular supplemental exercise. The most successful MotivateFit students are committed to supplemental exercise as part of their fitness lifestyle.

Types of Supplemental Exercise

There are two types of supplemental exercise that are critical for weight loss: cardio or aerobic exercise and strength training. Each type of exercise increases the body's expenditure of fuel ("burning" of calories). This helps to realign the energy imbalance of increased calories in, decreased calories out. Combining strength training with aerobic exercise is highly effective for weight loss, muscular development, and metabolism acceleration.

Aerobic Exercise is a cardio-respiratory activity that uses continuous, rhythmic large muscle group movements, which require the heart and lungs to work harder to meet the body's demand for oxygen. The increased demand upon the cardio-respiratory system causes an increased expenditure of calories.

Excess calories are stored in the body as fat. Achieving weight loss requires maximizing total caloric expenditure to achieve maximum fat utilization. Aerobic exercise is essential because it can be sustained long enough to expend a significant number of calories, thus becoming an effective weight loss activity.

Strength Training involves a variety of resistance exercises. Resistance exercises require the body's muscles to work or hold against an applied force. They increase muscle strength and bone integrity, and can sculpt the body with increased muscle definition. This is generally achieved through the use of weights, machines, and workout bands. Activities such as push-ups, sit-ups, and pull-ups are additional resistance exercises that utilize the body's own weight as a resistance.

Strength training results in an increase of lean body mass, which mainly consists of muscles. Because muscle expends more calories, even at rest (when compared to fat), it promotes an increase in RMR (resting metabolic rate). The increased RMR utilizes more calories and boosts the body's metabolism rate.

This supports your ability to lower and manage your weight.

Balance the F.A.T. in Your Physical Activity

Planning your exercise and physical activities requires you to balance the F.A.T. components: *frequency, amount and type.*

F (Frequency) applies to the number of days per week or number of times per day you will engage in exercise.

A (Amount) applies to either the amount of time or duration you will be engaged and/or the amount of intensity of the specific activity. The range of an activity's intensity may span from the least challenging to the most challenging, depending upon the specific activity or type of exercise and overall fitness.

T (Types of physical activity) are numerous and varied. Again, no *one* size fits all. But the most critical understanding of **T** (type), for increasing your physical activity, is that **T (type) will determine the F (frequency) and the A (amount).** The objective of whichever **T** (type) you choose remains constant. At the very minimum, the activity engaged in must be done regularly and for a minimum of fifteen to twenty minutes in order to have a demonstrable effect on fitness and weight loss.

The following four F.A.T. profiles for supplemental exercise are *balanced* and recommended for MotivateFit students. You should choose the profile that best suits your lifestyle. *Using the right F.A.T. balance supplemental exercise profile—you can make the progression from sedentary to very active in a safe, enjoyable, and effective way.*

1. **High frequency, low amount, different types**—an example would be going from relaxing yoga one day—to low intensity weight training the next day—to moderate aerobics the next day. Regardless of supplemental exercise intensity, you should always take at least one day off from exercise every week.

2. **Low frequency, high amount, and same type**—an example would be playing your favorite higher intensity sport once or twice a week.

3. **Low frequency, high amount, and different types**—an example would be engaging in different higher intensity exercise options (such as jogging and strength training) on two different days of the week (and not on consecutive days).

4. **High frequency, low amount, same type**—an example would be moderate, low impact aerobic exercise five to six days a week. Be sure you really enjoy the exercise chosen so that you can maintain motivation to stay consistent and avoid boredom.

The following four F.A.T. profiles for supplemental exercise are *imbalanced* and not recommended for MotivateFit students.

1. **High frequency, high amount, and same type**—this "overzealous" exercise profile will often lead to injury due to repetition of the same intense activity.

2. **High frequency, high amount, and different types**—this "overzealous" exercise profile will still lead to burnout because your body will not have time to recover from consecutive days of one intense activity to the next.

3. **Low frequency, low amount, and same type**—this "minimalist" exercise profile will have little or no impact on fitness, weight loss, and will often lead to boredom and declining motivation.

4. **Low frequency, low amount, and different type**—this second "minimalist" exercise

profile option has more variety, but will still have little or no impact on fitness and weight loss.

Warming up and Cooling Down

Whether your supplemental exercise intensity level is moderate or vigorous, do not neglect to warm up and cool down. Warm-up and cool-down periods are essential elements of any effective exercise program.

Warming up the muscles and connective tissue minimizes the risk of injury and prepares the heart and circulatory system for an increase in physical activity. Cooling down allows your heart rate, blood flow, and breathing to naturally return to normal. Immediately following cool-down is also the perfect time to engage in stretching and flexibility exercises, because the muscles are still warm.

It is also beneficial to drink plenty of water to prevent dehydration. Drink water before, during, and after vigorous exercise. Do not wait until you are thirsty. Be proactive and stay hydrated for optimal performance and results.

Chapter 9

Develop Your Fitness Habit

I enjoy helping others identify and develop new habits that will help them succeed and get better results in their life. The creation and formation of a powerful, life-changing habit—such as regular exercise--provides a more secure foundation for long-term fitness and weight loss success.

Your goal (as a MotivateFit student) is not just to develop a new habit. Rather, you will also focus on developing and mastering the actual *skill of developing and maintaining your fitness motivation.*

Below is an 8-step process for improving your *"fitness motivation skills."* Use this process to boost your fitness motivation, jumpstart your new fitness habit, and make the new habit "stick."

If you have been unable to develop the fitness habit in the past—you can use this proven process to help identify and implement the missing steps in your fitness plan or process.

Step 1: Clarify Your Motivation

The first step in creating your new fitness habit is to identify and strengthen the source of your motivation. Take the time to identify all motivators, including intrinsic (internal) and extrinsic (external) drivers. Personal fitness goals that align strongly with your values are great motivators. In addition, external pressures that push you toward needing the results from the fitness habit can act as fuel for intense motivation.

Don't hesitate to use the twin motivators of pleasure and pain to help increase your overall motivation for fitness and weight loss. The pleasure of the benefits from a habit will motivate most. However, the pain of the consequences from *not* mastering a habit can be a powerful motivator for many. It's okay to use fear to your advantage if it causes you to take productive action.

Step 2: Prioritize The Habit

Creating a new, life-changing habit is not easy. It takes mental and physical energy. In order to have sufficient energy to develop your new fitness habit—you must not overextend yourself with too many new goals or activities.

The secret is to focus on developing one significant habit at a time until you build momentum, and it starts to stick!

Avoid introducing unnecessary stress or new activities into your life during the formation of a significant habit. I understand that this is not always under your control, but my point is that you must control what you can so that you can conserve your energy for the creation of your vital fitness habit. It is a priority—right? If so—you should not have a problem prioritizing it (even it means eliminating something else from your life to make room).

Step 3: Focus on Frequency

Clarify your motivation. Prioritize your habit. Now, you must focus on frequency of the fitness habit. This is a critical step because it represents the essence of the habit formation process—creating the pattern of repeated behavior.

In order to focus on frequency, you must *not* allow yourself to become too concerned with unrelated factors, such as how long you engage in exercise or how intensely you engage in exercise. Remember—*focus on frequency*. This means that *you must engage in exercise daily until it becomes a habit*.

If this requires you to cut down the physical activity time or intensity—do it. You may start with 5 minutes of exercise daily. You can and should focus on increasing intensity and duration as you progress, but don't worry about this for now. You must commit to exercising daily in the beginning—in order for the psychological and physiological patterns to develop in your brain.

Step 4: Make It Easy

In addition to focusing on frequency, you must make sure exercise feels easy and simple--particularly in the early stages of new habit formation. If this means only one to five minutes of exercise—that's okay.

You know that your habit activity is easy enough if you finish wanting to do more or go longer. Resist this temptation! Making it easy is intentional. It helps accelerate the connections in your brain that accept the new activity as a pattern, and without internal resistance--which might not happen if you were to push yourself too hard too soon. Choose to work harmoniously with your brain—not against it, and it will reward you.

Step 5: Use Micro Goals

Most elite athletes and successful people need goals like most people need water. I, too, am a fanatical goal setter. So, for me, this step was initially a challenge.

As with most things, goals are effective for creating a new habit. However, my research and work with MotivateFit students has convinced me that goal setting must be approached in a specific manner when trying to instill a new significant habit in your life. That is—you must use "micro goals."

A micro goal is a very simple and near term objective. These are not the big vision or dream goals in the distant future. Big goals are motivating, but they are not as effective for new habit creation.

Micro goals are best designed to support the development of a new behavior pattern. It's not about the distant result, but more about the behavior—or, yes that's right—*the habit!*

The micro goal for new habit creation is <u>always</u> the same--*to do the habit activity on as many consecutive days as possible until it becomes a habit.* The *only* metric of success or failure is the number of consecutive days— period. *Your micro goal for fitness habit creation must be based on the duration of consecutive days*--and not based on work intensity or work results.

Step 6: Schedule It

The next logical step in the fitness habit creation process is to schedule the habit activity. Studies have concluded that scheduling an activity will double the probability of action.

By scheduling your exercise or fitness activity, you are consciously making time for it--and sending a strong signal to your brain and those around you that this is a priority. Guard this very small window of time very closely and do not let anything short of a dire emergency interfere with it.

Write or record your daily habit activity as a daily appointment or input it as a repeating task. You can use a smartphone, computer, tablet, or plain pen and paper. Just be sure to capture your daily habit activity somewhere that is convenient for you--so that you will have a daily reminder.

Step 7: Create Environmental Support

At this point in the process, most people are ready to get going on their new fitness habit activity. Not so fast. Trust me, it's worth working through the steps in sequential order—even if this means starting the new exercise a day or two later.

Creating a supportive environment will be less draining on your motivation and willpower. It will enable you in the fitness habit creation process.

Consider and address the following during this step:

*Inform and gain the support of your immediate family (remind them that it's not much time).

*Commit to getting adequate sleep (even if you have to eliminate a few non-essential activities).

*Purchase or acquire anything that is essential for your new exercise and fitness habit.

Step 8: Do It!

Okay—now it's time to actually start the new fitness habit. Simply put—it's time to *take action!*

This step in the process is precisely where you will really exercise your motivation. Don't worry--you will be able to take action consistently (daily) if you have followed the previous steps up to this point.

Some beginning MotivateFit students use self-talk or internal pep talks to get themselves going on their fitness habit activity each day. Others simply use a command or trigger—such as "let's go" or "let's do it." Use what works for you.

Ultimately, you will always come to that exact time in the day where you have to exercise (flex) your fitness motivation in the moment—and *take action to start the physical activity*. Do it!

Chapter 10

Enjoy Your Fitness Lifestyle

The following is a short story of one of my colleagues and his flawed relationship with fitness. He has allowed me to share this story with you.

David, known as Sgt. D., even by his civilian friends, is 38 years old and has been active military for eighteen years. He is married with a fifteen-year-old teenage son. Six days a week at 5 a.m., David runs five miles. He tries to get his son (David Jr.) to run with him, but D.J. is not about to get up any earlier than necessary to get to high school on time. D.J. loves his Dad, but thinks he is a hard-core nut. David loves his son but thinks he is soft and lazy.

"Son--*if you won't go running, at least get up and do some calisthenics, or go out to the weight bench in the garage and lift before school.*"

"*But, Dad, I'm not in the military. I don't play sports, so why would I do that?*"

David responds, saying--"*It's good discipline. It builds character. If you respect your body and challenge it to a higher level, it will always serve you.*"

D.J. retorted--"*I respect my body by letting it sleep, and by NOT feeding it raw eggs and forcing it to run up and down hills before dawn. My body is serving me just fine.*"

"*Eating breakfast burritos, lying around playing video games and sleeping half the morning away is not respecting your body,*" snapped David.

"*Getting up at 7 am is not sleeping half the morning away. How many other people do you see running around at 5 am?,*" says D.J.

"*Certainly not lazy people,*" says David—walking away just as his wife enters the room. David didn't want to hear his wife take their son's side again.

"*Leave him alone, David. D.J. just wants to go to school and have a little fun. He's a typical teenager,*" says David's wife.

"*Typically lazy,*" David thinks to himself. David doesn't understand why they just don't get it. Especially his son, for whom he has modeled fitness since the day he was born. How could *his* son not care about fitness as much as he did?

Unfortunately, I informed Davd that he doesn't realize just how wrong he is. He has *not* been modeling a modern fitness lifestyle. Far from it.

Yes, D.J. has seen his father's *interpretation* of what living a fit life is all about, and he wants no part of it. What D.J. sees is deprivation, restriction, a hard-nosed attitude, fanaticism, and absolutely no enjoyment. D.J. shrugs his shoulders, *"No pain, No gain? Is he kidding me? Where's the fun in that?"*

David has all the skills and habits, managing both his diet and his physical activity level--but he is so zealous about it that there is no enjoyment in the process. David, in fact, is "out of balance." He is the kind of guy you would want to go to war with you, but not to the gym for an enjoyable or motivating workout.

David's admirable fitness level is maintained as an obligatory chore that simply must be done and done his way. D.J. calls him "old school," because his Dad loves calisthenics—push ups, pull ups, rope climbing, and arm wrestling. Running, weight lifting, and exhausting calisthenics are viewed by David as the "old school" way to achieve physical fitness. He loathes high-tech exercise machines, modern day nutrition, yoga classes, aerobics, and variety or rest days as part of a fitness program. If injured or not feeling well, Sgt. D. believes you should just "suck it up" and push through it without taking a day off.

Sgt. D. means well. He is a great husband and father, but overbearing and relentless when it comes to his limiting view of a healthy diet and physical activity. He has accomplished much, yet will not celebrate his successes. Sgt. D's tunnel vision of maintaining health and fitness doesn't even allow for the possibility of having fun or enjoyment.

David is not living the MotivateFit lifestyle--or a balanced fitness lifestyle. Very few people will be motivated to stay fit or maintain this this distorted and unhealthy version of fitness if doing so makes them miserable and unhappy. Who could blame them? Just ask D. J.

There is a better way to get motivated for fitness—stay motivated for fitness—and enjoy the process along the way! By using the MotivateFit method--you can and will apply the correct knowledge, planning, resources, and skills to *get maximum long-term benefits and joy from minimum effort.*

Reject No Pain, No Gain

"No pain, no gain" is often cited as an inspirational quote to motivate and encourage persistence. The fallacy in this approach to fitness and weight loss is that it directly equates pain with progress and success.

Ironically--*avoiding pain* is a more natural and biologically wired human response and motivator.

It's true that you must challenge yourself in order to grow and develop the body and mind you are seeking. However, *challenges can be enjoyable*—whereas pain (despite being a vital and necessary human function) is simply not enjoyable.

Instead of seeking and fighting through the pain—I've found that it's much more motivating to reject this outdated notion of fitness and weight loss. As a MotivateFit student, you should do the same.

You can achieve your fitness and weight loss goals--live a healthy life—and not be miserable doing it (or like David—driving everyone else around you crazy). Fitness and weight loss do not have to be stressful.

The process of adopting a fitness lifestyle can be very motivating and fulfilling if you take the time to customize your program using MotivateFit elements, modern science, and natural laws.

Enjoyment is a proven ingredient in the successful achievement of fitness and weight loss goals. Enjoyment doesn't mean easy. Human bodies are meant to move. We are built for exercise and physical activity. Our bodies crave and need physical activity for living—this is why regular, proper exercise feels so good!

Your objective as a MotivateFit student is to develop a program and plan that allows you to fully *embrace and enjoy the physical, mental, and emotional benefits of regular exercise and a healthy diet.*

Once you have an ingrained fitness habit— your physical transformation is almost guaranteed. It will take a few weeks of dedicated focus to really find the perfect combination of activities and diet practices that work best for your body, mind, and lifestyle. But, you should give yourself credit and kudos for sticking with it. Do not beat yourself up just because you may falter along the way. Simply adjust and keep moving happily forward!

As a MotivateFit student, *you should always include "the joy" in your fitness and weight loss program.*

Do not engage in acts of desperation, deprivation, or pain for the sake of fitness or weight loss. Instead, design a healthy diet and exercise plan that will keep you fit *and* happy. Without the "joy" component of the equation, you are less likely to stay motivated and maintain the program.

Personalize Your Weight Loss

Personalization is the act of injecting yourself, on an intimate level, into the process. It requires a personal perspective and involvement. It promotes viewing your fitness or weight loss as "I, my, or mine." Your fitness or weight loss goal should be narrowly focused on your personal needs in the first person, and not as a "one size fits all" solution from an outside source.

You must make a conscious choice to personalize your fitness and weight loss plan for effectiveness and enjoyment.

Acknowledge and use the principle of personalization coupled with the five elements of MotivateFit (knowledge, planning, resources, actions, and skills) to accelerate the process of developing your fitness habit. This approach will allow you to cruise happily to your fitness and weight loss goals!

Program Yourself for Success

As you start to achieve your desired results—you will notice an increase in your confidence and self-esteem. Please be sure to internalize this sense of fulfillment at every step in your personal journey to fitness and weight loss.

Make this process of staying in touch with your "sense of success" a frequent habit. Congratulate yourself at every single step along the way in your exercise and healthy diet program. This self-recognition habit will "multiply your motivation" as you build your new fitness lifestyle.

Your basic mental encoding will determine a lot about how you perform and ultimately--how successful you will become in achieving your fitness goals. It is nearly impossible to overcome bad or negative programming unless you are conscious of the problem and have identified the root cause and solution.

The fact is--your thoughts, beliefs, and actions are largely determined by your programming. The good news is that this programming is well under your control. Consequently, you have the power and ability to program yourself for fitness and weight loss.

If you want to maximize your motivation and mind power—it is imperative that you take an active role in managing the programming of your mind. Without a high level of engagement in filtering and controlling your internal and mental programming—you will be hard pressed to achieve your innate fitness potential.

Highly fit individuals typically exhibit high levels of mental control. They believe that the mind is a precious commodity that must be protected and managed at all times. The best way to do this is through consistent programming and conditioning.

Mental programming for motivation, fitness, and weight loss success is possible through the following six methods:

1. Talking

2. Listening

3. Visualizing (imagining)

4. Viewing (seeing)

5. Feeling

6. Acting (taking action)

What you *say, hear, imagine, see, feel, and do* has a definite impact on your mental functioning and physical performance. If you control these methods-- you can control your mental programming. Programming that is aligned with (and supports) the realization of your fitness goals is good programming. On the contrary—bad programming (from you or an external source) will conflict with your fitness goals and prohibit long-term success.

The most important takeaway for you is to "be conscious" of programming at all times. Learn to pay very close attention to what you say, listen to, imagine, view, feel, and do as it relates to your body, weight, and fitness.

As you become more committed to the fitness lifestyle--programming for success and countering negative programming will become second nature and automatic.

It is very difficult to know if any communication or programming is positive or negative without first knowing your desired results and goals. Once you have clarity in your goals, it is easy to determine if incoming programming is beneficial or detrimental.

For example, if your goal is to become a national champion in your chosen sport—any programming that undermines effective training or game execution is negative programming. This might include a diet that is not balanced and nutritious—or not having the right conditioning program to support your fitness goals. Negative programming will prevent talented athletes from reaching their full potential in their sport.

Don't allow yourself to be programmed by negative people (better known as "drain people") or adverse circumstances. Don't invest time, attention, or energy into things that don't contribute to your goals and values. Keep your mind on lockdown against fitness or weight loss failure by exercising and applying your MotivateFit skills regularly.

Science has proven that conscious, positive, and productive mental programming leads to faster motivation development--which leads to mental control, better actions, and better results.

Keep in mind that programming yourself for success is not hard. It is just as easy as programming yourself for failure. In fact, programming yourself for failure is much more difficult because of the negative and damaging impact it can have on your life.

Don't be discouraged if you have allowed negative programming to sabotage your fitness or weight loss efforts in the past. You can reverse negative programming. The sooner you start increasing your MotivateFit capacity with more productive programming—the sooner you will start to see faster progress toward becoming a fitness and weight loss success.

Don't wait. Start using the principle of programming today! Make a solemn promise to yourself that you will never allow negative programming to infiltrate your mind.

With consistent and effective programming, the fitness mentality will transfer from your conscious mind to your subconscious mind where it will start to permeate your core beliefs and behaviors. This is a critical turning point, which will start your transformation into a committed fitness lifestyle practitioner with outstanding fitness motivation and discipline.

Eat for Pleasure

Committing to lifelong fitness and weight management does not mean that your life will forever be void of eating for pleasure. The key is that you must expand your taste experiences and learn to enjoy increased variety in your "palate paradise."

Try to insert something new into your healthy diet on a regular basis. There are hundreds of nutrient-dense and healthy foods that can be prepared in delicious and appetizing ways. Explore unfamiliar, yet healthier preparation options for your favorite dishes.

Many MotivateFit students have told me that they have expanded their diet options significantly after committing to the fitness lifestyle—because they are enjoying the journey of exploring new types of foods and recipes. In studies--*a personalized, healthy, and constantly expanding diet has proven to be much more satisfying and enjoyable when compared to a common, unhealthy, and limited diet.*

Prepare for dining. Make it a mini event and experience. Avoid the practice of "grab and go" eating. Savor the experience by eating slowly. Allow your palate to familiarize itself with something a bit different. You may discover a new favorite.

Approach every meal as a good thing that supports your commitment to achieving your important fitness and weight loss goals. If your goals are important—then taking the time to engage in regular exercise and healthy eating must also become important in your life.

Become a healthy-eating connoisseur and seek out information about fine, gourmet, healthy eating. Healthy eating does not have to be bland, boring and tasteless. Set out to prove that point.

On those occasions when you have made a conscious decision to eat an old favorite, such as your favorite chocolate or desert, and not for fuel--but simply for pleasure, just remember to *keep the balance*. When the T (type) is slightly less than the optimum healthy choice, adjust A (the amount or portion size and) F (the frequency of those occasions).

Using your MotivateFit skills and fitness lifestyle habits—you can confidently indulge in a healthy way by not treating the occasional decadent snack as a feast or last meal.

Exercise for Pleasure

Exercise does not have to be drudgery—a chore that must be endured. Moderate or vigorous physical activity can produce endorphins that promote a pleasurable experience. This experience is often referred to as being "in the *flow* or *zone*." Many have experienced the zone—a physical and psychological state of hyper-focus and pleasure.

Those who engage in regular physical activity have experienced the effects of *the flow* first hand. They report feelings of intense focus and concentration, confidence, energized effort, and an awareness of pleasure. They literally feel psychologically in flow with their physical activity.

Learn to recognize, connect with, and enjoy the occurrence of flow within your own exercise and physical activity experiences.

You can promote increased enjoyment during exercise by listening to your favorite music—and by focusing on keeping your breathing and body relaxed.

Utilize your exercise experience as an opportunity to socialize and reduce stress. If it helps and fits your personality—try to make exercise a competitive game, or simply choose sports that you enjoy.

Always conclude your exercise sessions on a high note or when you are feeling invigorated! Avoid exercising to the point of feeling drained and tired. You want to end your exercise sessions "in the zone." If you stop while you are still wanting more—you will come back the next time raring to go! This pattern will strengthen your fitness motivation over time.

Celebrate Your Success

The secret to staying motivated for fitness and weight loss is enjoying the journey every step of the way. As you achieve milestones (no matter how small) along the way to your ultimate fitness goals—I encourage you to celebrate your success. *Success happens in small steps before it can happen in long miles.*

Focus on congratulating yourself constantly and developing happy feelings connected to the fact that you are treating your body well, getting results, and growing your motivation skills. Celebrate your unique fitness and weight loss journey—short term and, at the destination, long term. But don't celebrate every single victory with a large chocolate fudge sundae! Instead, over time, success itself will become the most enjoyable reward—which will only increase your fitness motivation.

Expand Your Circle of Success

I encourage you to develop a fitness lifestyle circle of friends, family, and supporters. Focus on connecting with those who have achieved success, experts who can help you achieve success, and those who share a similar desire to achieve their fitness and weight loss goals.

Be sure to allow those who have encouraged and supported you to be a part of your key celebrations and milestones.

As you become more fit and motivated, it will increase your commitment if you will "pay it forward" by supporting others who are trying to achieve their fitness and weight loss goals. Share your experiences, failures, and successes with your circle.

Don't forget to seize opportunities to put your increasing fitness and energy into action by participating in more social physical activities.

Try reconnecting with the child in you. Remember playing? You engaged in tag, skipping, jumping, hopping, running, and tumbling—all physical activities that provided the child in you with the proper exercise that was needed. You didn't set out to exercise; you went out to play. Exercise and social connecting were merely byproducts of playing.

Recall those feelings and experiences of playing. Shift your perception from exercise participation as work or a duty and *make the transition to physical fun or play*. Have fun; go find some friends and play!

Chapter 11

Maintain Your Fitness and Weight Loss

As a MotivateFit student, you are able to eat healthy and exercise on regular basis. You do not make excuses, but instead make decisions—and take the necessary actions. Consequently, you are making progress toward your fitness and weight loss goals.

Using the MotivateFit elements—you can develop the skills, habits, and commitment to lead an enjoyable fitness lifestyle. Lasting fitness and weight loss requires that you do not abandon the process and routines that led to your current success.

Losing weight and getting fit is challenging; maintaining fitness and weight loss can be more challenging if you are not equipped with the proper knowledge. Some people are able to achieve a moderate level of weight loss or fitness success, but very few are able to maintain their success long-term.

My goal is to help you join the celebrated few who are able to stay consistently motivated to maintain their fitness and weight management programs as part of their daily life.

Launch, Connect, Cruise

In my experience working with athletes, fitness enthusiasts, and weight loss seekers—I've come to realize that there are essentially three phases of success on the journey to a successful fitness lifestyle and permanent weight loss.

1. Launch Phase

2. Connect Phase

3. Cruise Phase

Launch

In the launch phase, you start the process of gathering information, making decisions, and taking initial action steps to achieve your fitness and weight loss goals.

The key to success in this phase is to be patient and take the time to address and develop each individual MotivateFit element. Most people who fail to stay motivated and achieve their fitness goals are not willing to follow the proven steps to success.

Connect

In the connect phase, you have started making changes in your daily life. You are eating healthier and exercising more regularly. You are starting to see positive changes in your body--your motivation is high—and you are gaining confidence.

The key to success in this phase is to avoid letting inevitable setbacks keep you from moving forward. You will have setbacks. Prepare for it by committing to always get back on track after a setback—and learn to utilize your support network.

Successful MotivateFit students understand that a setback is an indication that you need to change something in your plan, decision-making, or actions. Stay positive, smart, and keep going forward toward your fitness and weight loss success!

Cruise

In the final cruise phase, you have fully adopted a fitness lifestyle, and you are "cruising" to your fitness and weight loss goals. You are easily able to maintain your healthy diet and exercise habits.

As this stage—you are fully engaged in the MotivateFit method—and your physical transformation seems to be happening on semi-autopilot, because you are enjoying the process and results. As you continue to cruise—the weight continues to come off--and you feel stronger, more energetic, more relaxed, and more focused.

By the cruise phase, you will be a MotivateFit master student—you will be living a fitness lifestyle-- and you will be able to easily resist any temptations from fitness fantasyland.

Continue to hone your fitness motivation by staying engaged with all of the MotivateFit elements. *Consistent use of all MotivateFit elements (knowledge, planning, resources, actions, and skills) will help you maintain peak motivation for fitness.*

Solutions for Setbacks

The following strategies and tips will help you maintain your fitness motivation, exercise habits, and healthy diet patterns.

Clear Objectives

Having clear objectives allows you to track and measure your progress. Without clear objectives, your actions will be less productive. With clear objectives, you will see and feel progress—and real growth provides added motivation to continue improving. Don't underestimate the power of clarity!

I recommend using the S.M.A.R.T. method of goal setting to help bring clarity, power, and inspiration to your objectives. The S.M.A.R.T. acronym is broken down as follows:

S–Specific (focus the goal on a specific area; for example—weight loss or strength gains)

M–Measurable (quantify the goal or at least clarify the key indicator of progress; for example--the number of consecutive days of exercise—or the number of times throughout the day that willpower was successfully exercised to resist unhealthy diet thoughts and impulses)

A–Actionable (an action-oriented goal is more effective because you can actually *do something* to achieve it)

R–Realistic (make sure the goal is attainable with reasonable, consistent action)

T–Timed (quality goals typically specify *when* the desired result will be achieved)

Use the S.M.A.R.T. goal setting method to fine-tune your objectives. It is worth the small investment of time.

I have two tips when it comes to goal setting.

1. *Avoid having too many goals at one time.* Strive for 1-3 specific fitness or weight loss goals. I have found

that having fewer goals allows me to focus and progress much faster. If my goal is to increase improve my diet --I will be 100% committed to this until I reach my S.M.A.R.T. goals.

2. *Use "Skill Stacking."* Don't try to maximize all of your MotivateFit elements at the same time. Instead, focus on improving one specific element (e.g. knowledge) until you start gaining momentum—and then move on to developing the next element. Use skill stacking and habit stacking to ensure consistent progress.

Regular Reviews

You have just finished a great workout. You are in the zone and you can feel the improvement in your motivation, stamina, and strength.

So, what's next? Well, for starters--don't simply disengage until the next workout. Between workouts--you should review your progress and make necessary adjustments to your program as needed.

Regular performance reviews are an integral part of all world-class organizations. Organization YOU can benefit from this proven tool for success. Superstar professional athletes have access to sophisticated equipment and dedicated personnel for this phase of their training program. You really don't need expensive tools or a bevy of assistant coaches— but you do need to *review your fitness and weight loss program regularly for continuous improvement.*

I have watched many people break through previous plateaus and elevate their MotivateFit skills to new, higher levels after getting serious about workout and diet reviews. I'm sure you will do the same. It only requires ten to fifteen minutes of your time.

MotivateFit Journal

A fitness journal is an indispensable tool for any athlete or MotivateFit student. With the help of a fitness journal--you can eliminate unproductive activity--and increase the focus on activities and strategies that are delivering the greatest improvements and results.

What you actually record in your training journal is up to you. It depends on your S.M.A.R.T. goals and the specific elements of the MotivateFit Method that you are concentrating on developing. I suggest keeping your notes simple and short--so that you will actually do it (record progress) regularly.

Information in my MotivateFit journal includes the following: date of the workout, current weight, MotivateFit element focus, workout duration, training tool or activity, progress on key metrics, diet selections, and relevant comments (suggestions for improvement, general observations, etc.)

You can choose to use a paper journal or digital journal on your smartphone (or computer). The key is to be consistent and accurate in your program reviews. Personally, I like to conduct my fitness program reviews immediately after a workout. I have found that this works best for me because I am typically feeling great and excited about my progress, which makes the review process more enjoyable and sustainable.

Body Awareness

In addition to using journals--you must *tune into your instincts for subconscious fitness and training guidance.* I am always amazed by the breakthrough solutions and answers I receive when I am attuned to my body, mind, and emotions.

Always listen closely to your body and mind for signals to push harder or hold back in your workouts—and for signs that perhaps you should make adjustments in your diet or sleeping habits. Develop heightened body and mind awareness. You will improve faster, maintain motivation, and avoid setbacks due to injuries or burnout.

Forgive Yourself

Prevention is the best way to avoid significant setbacks, but it's not foolproof. Setbacks will happen. It happens to all of us. Your goal should be to *minimize the time and impact of any setback*. Having proven solutions to help you recover and maintain your motivation will keep you on track to your fitness goals.

Above all else—don't let temporary setbacks get you down or make you feel guilty. Make decisions and take action to get back on track as soon as possible. Don't let one mistake cause you to spiral into a long phase of inactivity or disengagement. Understand that *you have the power to make a complete change every day*!

Self-Talk

As soon as you realize that you are indeed experiencing a setback, stop and have a brief talk with yourself. Acknowledge the setback and your feelings of disappointment. Recall your motivation foundation. Allow the setback to motivate you. Get the lesson of the setback. What occurred and why?

Internalize the lesson to break the negative cycle or downward spiral.

Forgive yourself and move forward, keeping in mind that you deserve to treat yourself better. You are a MotivateFit master student and you are simply experiencing a temporary setback that you will overcome.

Despite whatever else is going on in your life, know that you can keep your commitment to fitness in the midst of it. Allow that commitment to help you regain balance and self-confidence during stressful times, and steer you back to your fitness and weight loss goals.

Get Back on Track

Having identified the cause or causes of a temporary setback—you should commit immediately to "stopping the slide." Stop the unbalanced actions that are causing the regression and weight-gain by addressing the specific reason for the setback in the most direct and simple way. The goal is to "rebalance" and regain your motivation by disengaging from anything that is compromising your fitness progress (including your own thoughts, beliefs, actions, or drain people with negative programming or influencing).

Stay aware of potential pitfalls as you build your fitness motivation and fitness habits. The following factors can derail your fitness and weight loss progress.

Lack of Time

Lack of time or ineffective time management causes stress due to unhealthy overload in activity. Take a moment to reevaluate your priorities. Do not simply accept that there is not enough time. Make time in your schedule for fitness by giving up something that is less important or less urgent.

Lack of Sleep

Sleep deprivation disrupts the body's energy levels and depletes your willpower and motivation. Try to maintain a consistent sleep schedule that allows for adequate sleep. Your body needs sleep to recover from your physical workouts. The benefit of exercise and a fitness lifestyle is that it will help you sleep better by relaxing your body.

Emotional Overload

Stress can be very disruptive to your fitness motivation, healthy diet, and exercise consistency. To counter the effects of stress, try the following:

*Use your social circles to help resolve minor stress related to daily challenges.

*Re-connect to your goals to help maintain focus on what's most important.

*Learn not to sweat the small stuff by learning to "let go" of minor stressors. Save your mental energy for your major goals, including fitness and weight loss.

*Try meditation to recharge your mind and rebalance emotions.

*Try exercise or go for a leisurely walk with a friend. Physical activity is a proven stress buster.

*If you have experienced a significant emotional trauma, please seek out the help of a healthcare professional.

New or transitional life events--such as moving, marriage, career change, new baby, or the death of a close family member will definitely alter established routines and behaviors. Understand that some things will take a temporary back seat and plan for this. Re-shift your priorities, but do not abandon a regular healthy diet and regular effective physical activity, even if you have to adjust the type of exercise or foods.

If you allow yourself to be flexible and open to making the necessary adjustments to your exercise and diet routines—you can make it through significant life events without losing your fitness level or gaining weight. Be sure to stay connected to family and friends to help maintain mental and emotional health during these challenging times.

Injury or illness

First and foremost—you should follow your doctor's advice when dealing with any serious injury or illness. Take it slow. Your body's number one priority is healing itself. Maintain a healthy diet and lower your calorie intake to compensate for the temporary lack of physical activity and the sedentary consequences of the illness or injury. Be sure you are cleared to resume physical activity before proceeding with your exercise program. Remember, basic health comes before fitness.

Joyful Events

Holiday gatherings, vacations, and birthday celebrations are common causes of temporary fitness derailments. There are things you can do to minimize the effect.

Drink plenty of water throughout the invent to minimize liquid calories and sugar. If you want to eat a variety of tasty foods—try eating a balanced meal before the event so that you are able to eat smaller portions during the event. Drink alcohol in moderation—and if you are drinking alcohol, consider having a glass of water between each drink.

Don't go on a guilt trip. Relax and enjoy the event. Commit that you will exercise the next day to make up for the indulgence.

Failure Triggers

Personal failure triggers--such as emotional eating, relationship stress, or business travel can be especially challenging. The first step is to know and understand your unique triggers. The second step is to develop proactive plans and strategies to mitigate your personal failure triggers so that they don't cause you to spiral into an extended period of unhealthy eating and physical inactivity.

Do not ignore or underestimate your personal triggers. Stay aware and continue to gain the knowledge and skills necessary to counter the triggers and continue making progress. Seek out additional help from friends, family, and (if necessary) professionals.

Whenever you are facing a negative trigger event—you can override and weaken the trigger by continuously affirming your commitment to the fitness lifestyle (through words, decisions, and actions).

Conclusion

Final Thoughts on Fitness Motivation

Congratulations! You have completed the study of fitness motivation for weight loss, exercise, and sports.

For fast results, start incorporating the information in this book into your daily life. Apply the relevant principles of fitness motivation and utilize the MotivateFit™ method and process.

You will be delighted by the increase in your motivation for fitness, exercise, healthy eating, and weight loss—the improvement in your habits and consistency--and the transformation in how you look, feel, and perform.

Reading this book will not turn you into a champion athlete or provide you with the greatest physique in world. However, if you use the information, principles, and drills as instructed--you will increase your fitness motivation and develop a sustainable fitness habit in your daily life. Consistent application of the information contained in this guide is guaranteed to maximize your fitness motivation and help you reach your fitness and weight loss goals.

By covering one specific success skill, fitness motivation, in detail--my goal is to keep this book distinguished and highly regarded. My mission is to maintain the highest standard of quality on this topic by providing information that is simple, affordable, innovative, and highly effective in helping you achieve your fitness and weight loss goals.

--C. Townsend

Thank You

My sincere thanks to you for purchasing and reading this book. If you are satisfied with this book, please take a moment to leave a helpful review on Amazon.

Your feedback is greatly appreciated, and it will help me continue to write books that help you get results and achieve your fitness and weight loss goals.

Made in the USA
Middletown, DE
08 July 2019